To H. & J.,

In memory of wounding and healing,
healing and wounding again.

Table of Content

10
I On Optimisation, PMDD and its Metaphors

28
II The Internet is the Recipe: Sexual and Psychological Education in Digital Spheres

46
III Elevated and Upgraded: The Paradigms of Female Health and Body Optimisation

60
IV Gathering the Wounded Traces: From Self-Study to Data Collections

V FemTech: Discourse, Surveillance, and Privacy 76

VI Predictive Healing: On the Use of Algorithms in FemTech Apps 92

VII The Glitch Ideology and the Potentiality of Contingency with Carmen Hines 112

Acknowledgments 124

Bibliography

Introduction

In 2020, I couldn't count the days I was able to function. Every new month seemed clearly and distinctly divided into two: the first part, where I could behave, function, and perform the individual I promised to be. The second part, in which I was a failing piece of flesh holding myself together with the loose bits of me remaining. On a metro in Amsterdam, I recall telling my partner at the time that if this is how some people feel all the time, I understand why someone would want to die. Yet overall, nothing was wrong. I was lacking sleep, stressed and scared, but other than that, life was pretty much bearable. I had no specific diagnosis, no particular way to explain to doctors what was going on with me. It was difficult to believe because the pain wasn't constant, and there were brief periods when I could see a blue sky, clear as day, before getting struck down, yet again, by another thunderstorm.

I remember vividly the first time I googled 'desperate two weeks out of four'. With such a strange prompt, the odds that I would find answers were thin and scarce. But, after a few hours of strolling, I found out that other people had phrased their issues in a similar way. This diagnosis, whatever it was, sounded like the strangest kind of war. It's deeply soothing yet also haunting to figure out what exactly is causing your body harm.

As a cis-woman with irregular periods and a messy hormonal life, I've been used to being confronted with a medical system that doesn't really understand my body from a very young age. From amenorrhea to irregular bleeding, chronic cystic inflammation to potential endometriosis diagnosis, I had to, like many others, educate myself and learn more about my body through searches and queries. Online, I discovered a community of individuals willing to share and learn from one another. There, I also realised that my experience was not uncommon, nor was it unique. The internet and its devices were my saviours, my delighted supporters.

The relationship between female bodies and the concept of technology isn't an intuitive one. Nevertheless, there's a long history of techno-feminism and cyber-feminism embracing precisely the possibilities technological changes hold and the potential resources and shared experiences on the internet. In my daily practice, I am the first to advocate for such things: growing up as a millennial, I seem to remain forever fascinated by the technological tools that came into existence during my childhood. Seduced by the power of virtuality, as a kid, I often caught myself hoping that I did not have a body. I frequently dreamt of not having to partake with its envelope, simply because it's so damn sweet sometimes not to experience the failures of my own flesh. Nowadays, I live in a constant dissonance, one where I experience empowerment from digital experiences while also seeing the deeply problematic issues that lie underneath the digital agenda. If I wrote this book, it is not because I despise technology. On the contrary: it is precisely because I believe in its liberating and transformative power that I want to participate in a critical reflection on existing tools, how they function, how they can be altered.

I recall the excitement I had when I first started writing about the topic of female health and technology. It felt like I had finally found a way to investigate the workings behind a long-lasting personal way of relating to my own body. A way to investigate something I believed to be 'dysfunctional'. I started this project to better understand these questions, while also collecting an assemblage of writers and thinkers who could help me dissect this research. In this book, I hope to give substantive resources to the reader while simultaneously rendering valid discourse around a topic I initially had a hard time navigating and researching myself. Technology in itself is not responsible for all the oppressive and normative structures that surround us. Instead, they result from our desire to compromise on our well-being in the wake of optimisation and perfection. What is the relationship between female bodies and technological progress? How is the lack of knowledge in female health and menstruating bodies rendered within the daily design of our technological society? How are certain recently developed technologies mirroring (past) conditioning of our bodies? Such questions could not have been investigated without interdisciplinary research and connections, as it seemed impossible to try to make sense of this phenomenon any other way. The result of this ongoing research, *Cycles, the Sacred and the Doomed*, is a book where the reader travels between philosophical and mythical concepts. From studying the internet as an open-source platform for holistic knowledge to a more in-depth analysis of the promises of FemTech technologies, this project attempts to display all the challenges and promises at hand in the tech-meets-female-body era. For this, I decided to intertwine personal experiences and auto-ethnography with theory. In doing so, I hope to bring a more empirical and sensitive approach to female health and its relation to technology: a way of researching that fits its at times soft, at times hard topic.

While this introduction is an opportunity for me to express my vision, it is also a chance to acknowledge my position on this topic as a cis-woman, as well as white and raised in a privileged environment. When writing from the 'I' perspective, I'm talking about personal experiences; when using 'we', I envision all menstruating and female bodies and women at large that surround me, those who are going through similar concerns. While this book mainly focuses on the lived experience of a cis-woman,

I want to acknowledge all bodies and genders that refer to the female; be they woman, non-binary, or trans—all of their laughter, all of their pain. You'll notice that I use both 'female bodies' and 'menstruating bodies', or even simply 'our bodies' when referring to this inclusive group of people, something that has been done from a practical sense of view, rather than an excluding one. Furthermore, I appreciate the positivity and care put into (female health) research, science, and technology—into our bodies—and recognise the workers behind these projects. I acknowledge all the individuals who have fought for women's rights, birth control, and abortion rights, the ones who still today fight for hormone therapy, and, generally, for more inclusive, free healthcare. I wish to write in memory of all the individuals, all genders included, who, for centuries, have been called hysteric, crazy, bipolar, on edge, insane, who have felt displaced, inadequate, alienated from their bodies, and severely misdiagnosed. I want to acknowledge all the past witches and healers, who have tried to calm our pain and suffering, who surely envisioned a future in which the technologies of our bodies would be fully embraced and somehow healed.

We're on our way.

Chapter I

On Optimisation, PMDD and its Metaphors

We must know whether we want to change the world to experience it with the same sensorial system like the one we already possess, or whether we'd rather modify our body, the somatic filter through which it passes.
– Excerpt from *Testo Junkie* by Paul B. Preciado

I woke up earlier than Juli, my partner. It's day fifteen. The fog is slowly appearing around me. I can't see it yet, but I feel and hear it. This hushed, cynical voice in my head, telling me that every attempt at fighting it is pointless. The slowly escalating anxiety rushing through my veins once I start to focus on what could go wrong. Right now, the sun's rays are slowly piercing through the mosquito net. My partner is still sleeping. The image of my parents pops up in my head: the bizarre idea of their monogamy and the strange concept of sleeping in the same bed night after night. I recall believing that the absence of consistency in relationships would be the definitive evidence of not being loved. Lying in bed, the thought alone of endless continuity and availability feels like a weight, a terrible pressure.

In her book *Illness as a Metaphor*, Susan Sontag investigates the cultural and aesthetic representations of disease in society. She explains how they are often displayed as images or meanings, instead of being seen as what they fundamentally are: a burden. A condition to be treated.[1] When I first started to research the term *Premenstrual Dysphoric Disorder*, better known as PMDD, I read its list of symptoms to see what it entailed. What a surprise and a relief when I realised that the diagnosis of such a condition was not purely scientific, but rather empirically based. Still, I wondered, how does one treat an ailment as a disease, when pain and discomfort are, in essence, seen as a fundamental component of our lives—at least, that is, as far as female bodies are concerned? Or so we are told.

PMDD existed as a metaphor before it was even categorised as a disease. Nowadays, it's a symbol of how the female body is treated and the prejudice around it. More than a disease, it results from the limited understanding of the effect hormones have on the body, psyche, and social life. PMDD shows us how one's body is seen in society.

1 Susan Sontag, *Illness as a Metaphor* (New York: Farrar Straus & Giroux, 1978).

Only once we understand the role this metaphor plays, and how it limits the possibilities for treatment, can we understand what's at stake behind the acknowledgment of such menstrual conditions.

Irritability. Nervousness. Lack of control. Agitation. Anger. Insomnia. Difficulty in concentrating. Depression. Severe fatigue. Anxiety. Confusion. Forgetfulness. Poor self-image. Paranoia. Emotional sensitivity. Crying spells. Moodiness. Trouble sleeping. Abdominal cramps. Bloating. Constipation. Nausea. Vomiting. Pelvic heaviness or pressure. Backache, Decreased coordination. Painful menstruation. Diminished sex drive. Appetite changes. Food cravings. Hot flashes....

Upon reading this list, one of the first things that comes to mind is: *'Whose menstruating body doesn't suffer from any of these?'* Naturally, severity and frequency vary from one individual to another. But still. PMDD is a floating cloud that englobes an entire field of dysfunctional behaviour and physical incapabilities. If you menstruate and feel terrible two weeks out of four, you likely have this condition, too. A complex one to diagnose, for sure, as the symptoms can be so diverse. As far as scientific knowledge goes, PMDD is generally understood as a dysfunctional reaction of the body from the change of hormones (here, progesterone and oestrogen) throughout the month, which is why symptoms usually disappear at the beginning of each cycle, when menstruation actually starts.

PMDD can be quite convoluted to study and diagnose. It regroups symptoms that can be dealt with individually, yet as a whole, turns into the impossibility of a human being to function.[2] Understanding the severity of this problem—female bodies barely being able to perform, yet its reasons barely researched—is too complex to grasp in a world where one is conditioned to think 'pain is normal' and 'menstruation is a curse one must suffer from in silent obedience'. A body suffering from such symptoms can hardly express what it is going through in a society that upholds the narrative—and has been for centuries—that being born with a uterus means complying to endure all of this. But still. Data collected demonstrates that 20 % of menstruating bodies deal with PMDD.[3] That's approximately 600,000,000 individuals. PMDD is a fluctuation one could, perhaps, deal with if we existed in a society that didn't value endless efficiency and competition so highly, or one that didn't see uteruses as objects deemed constantly available. Or even, if we dare to dream, one in which fair rates in the working environment exist, and generic medicine looks into causes, not just symptoms. Currently, PMDD is primarily being voiced and amplified online, resonating within the realm of unrecognised and misdiagnosed conditions.

2 Kate Lucey, "PMDD Is the Condition That Means Your Period Can Make You Suicidal," *Metro*, 2019.

3 Megan Hull, "Premenstrual Dysphoric Disorder Statistics," *The Recovery Village* (blog), May 8, 2023.

Those who suffer from PMDD are moralised, not only by the medical field but also by the people surrounding them. Perhaps their mental confusion is understood as hysteria, their low libido a lack of love, their frigidity a mystery. Perhaps their fluctuations are even seen as instability and their emotional 'unsustainability' as some sort of craziness. But let there be no confusion: PMDD is a condition, *a disease*, and a proper dysfunction. Like many other diseases, its effects are highly enhanced by its unrecognition, the absence of knowledge on the subject, and its confrontation with society's norms and values. Although the origins, triggers, and aggravating factors of the condition remain elusive, employing PMDD as a metaphorical concept provides a valuable perspective to examine technologies tailored for menstruating bodies and the progress made in this domain.

Many would argue that, over the course of the past century, enormous breakthroughs have been made in female health research. They would comment that the era of men sniffing menstrual blood and running away scared while the smoke of yet another female witch fills the air is, thankfully, long gone. And while I do agree with these statements, this by no means entails that the gender bias in medicine and research has been resolved. The majority of medical studies look into conditions from a *male* perspective, and, most commonly, women's studies remain poorly funded. It's time to dive into the depths and history of female bodies, taking a unique chance to gain a deeper understanding of the power dynamics and oppressive forces underlying most recent developments.

The Insufficient Technology of the Body

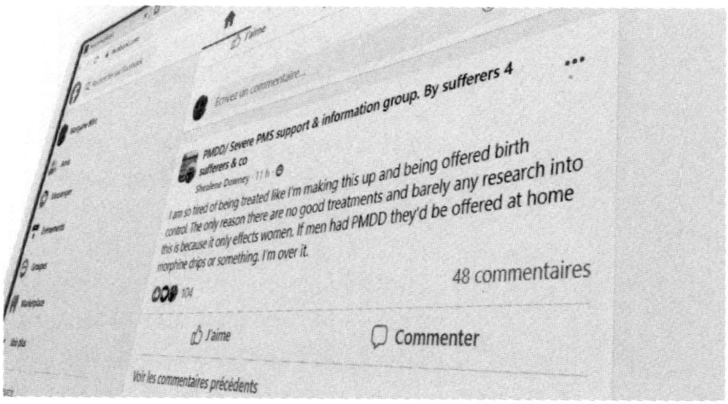

Figure 1 Screenshot from the Facebook group PMDD/Severe PMS Support, posted by Shealene Downey.

Female bodies and technologies have an ambiguous relationship. The ability to be fertile and grant *life* remains one of the biggest possibilities of human existence. For some, menstruation, the absence of menstruation, and the numerous fluctuations throughout our menstrual cycle are inherent technologies that foster self-awareness and awareness of our surroundings. This unique aspect of female bodies holds significant political implications (*danger!*). As a result, these bodies have been presented with various options, pills, supplements, and devices, all marketed as 'progress' to enhance the so-called optimal functioning of our bodies. As a human-lived technology, the body fluctuates and sometimes does not offer the best living experience. Not all bodies with the potential to menstruate actually do, or have a regular cycle. Not all of them ovulate or can conceive. Some struggle with intense pain; some are never able to experience pleasure. As previously emphasised, living with your initial biological condition does not mean living a better life: the workings of our bodies can affect various areas of life in quite unpleasant ways.

This past century, the advancements and pills proposed to us, menstruating bodies, held the promise of overcoming pain, obstacles, failures, and many other conditions. For the body's *accessibility*, birth control was provided. For the body's *reproductivity*, IVF. For the body's *longevity*, hormone replacement. Mental instability? Antidepressant. Unknown patterns and body fluctuations? Health and Menstruating Apps. The list goes on and on. While these technologies, initially seen as tools for both emancipation and freedom, used to bring out a lot of enthusiasm in female and menstruating communities, they are now seriously questioned and decked out with ethical, political, and ecological implications. This is particularly the case for individuals suffering from Polycystic Ovarian Syndrome (PCOS) or the aforementioned Premenstrual Dysphoric Syndrome (PMDD).[4] Although these two illnesses differ, they both reflect a similar issue: the body ails from its own technology, and the solutions provided are often inadequate. The result? Feelings of being misunderstood, of not being listened to. A valid reason for these communities to meet and share knowledge on digital platforms, such as Facebook, Reddit, or Instagram. But can internet support alone be the cure? Surely not. Still, these spaces demonstrate and underline the menstrual and medical revolution we are facing, as well as its complexities. With or without the pill, with or without these bodily conditions, our bodies are gradually realising that the environment in which we roam is not, by definition, *designed* for us. A problem that neither the pill, antidepressants, nor this false promise of optimality can hide any longer.

If these conditions are indeed a representation of our 'failed technology', recent studies which looked into the hormonal and social roots of PMS, universally known or experienced as premenstrual syndrome, demonstrated that its symptoms are highly impacted by the social environment one exists in. Many researchers have indeed investigated how its effects changed depending on the social environment, demonstrating how menstruating bodies, when failing to be super-efficient and adequate, often fall into self-pathologization:

4 Amy Leisner and Marissa Pomerance, "This Disorder Affects Millions Of Women, And No One is Talking About it. Why?," *The Candidly*, 2021.

'When women were able to be alone, they reported that their premenstrual symptoms were reduced; the "PMS" effectively disappeared, and they felt "better". However, many of the women we interviewed never took time out for themselves in the whole month, and spent little time engaged in leisure activities, focusing instead on the needs of others, common to women who present with "PMS" clinically.'[5]

5 Jane M. Ussher, "The Ongoing Silencing of Women in Families: An Analysis and Rethinking of Premenstrual Syndrome and Therapy," *Journal of Family Therapy* 25, no. 4 (2003).

Such perspectives on the subject can make us wonder: what is it that makes these bodies so-called inadequate in the first place? What sort of reference do we uphold when determining how we should function? While the conditions mentioned earlier (PCOS, PMDD, among others) are often grounded in physical and hormonal dysfunction, they seem to offer us a critical lens perfect for studying how our technological bodies are perceived and function. What solutions are being offered to us? Are these new tricks, pills and technologies actually helping menstruating bodies feel better and *heal* within society?

In her thesis, *The Genesis of Premenstrual Syndrome*, Bianca Zietal reinforces the idea of PMS as a social construct by illustrating how: *'the concept of PMS was developed and informed by the discovery of hormones and the resulting field of endocrinology that provided a framework for conceptualizing PMS.'*[6] Zietal expands her theory and demonstrates the metaphor of PMS illustrating its own unrecognition: *'This variety of uses suggests that popular culture understands PMS as something that makes for a good joke or serves to explain a negative change in a woman's behavior. However, relatively few people know that PMS has an official place as a medical diagnosis.'*[7] As she underlines in her text, it is precisely because we believe mood swings, pain, or mental disability are 'fundamental' aspects of menstruating bodies that, as a result, this well-known, seriously disabling phenomenon isn't properly addressed as such. By limiting the urgency and despair in their experiences, these bodies' needs are repressed, even repressing themselves in return.

Science alone won't help us. To just call out hormones and biological dysfunction as the sole cause of our displacement would be to deny certain societal constructs and the role they play. Through the lens of the condition of Premenstrual Dysphoric Disorder, manifesting as an intense collection of PMS, we can ask ourselves: how can PMDD help dissect and reconfigure the technologies of our bodies? Furthermore, how are these technologies taken care of in our society? More than just a chemical or hormonal imbalance, PMDD can be seen as a metaphor for our body's inadequacy. Yet could it also be the externalisation of our incapacity to fit so-called correctly into the puzzle of ideal 'efficiency'?

Today, we can scarcely find literature that addresses the topic of women and their mental illnesses. If we do, it's often written by the women themselves, who dare to ask the most urgent questions based on their own understanding and experiences. In *Women and Madness*,

6 Zietal, Bianca. "Thesis: The Genesis of Premenstrual Syndrome (PMS)," in: *Embryo Project Encyclopedia*, 2021.

7 Zietal, "The Genesis of Premenstrual Syndrome," 2021.

Jane Ussher expands on how her mother's condition drove her to study psychology and investigate the dynamics that go hand in hand with the pathologisation of women's dysfunctionality. There, Ussher borrows Caplin's following statement: *'In anofficial announcement nearly half of all Americans experience a psychatric disorder. Does that mean no one is normal? Or do we live in such a crazy-making, sick, impersonal society that it does serious psychological damage to half of us? Should we be calling women the mentally ill or society's wounded?'*[8] Let's take this realisation and apply it to the criteria and expectations of our Western culture, which lead to severe aggravation of our health.

8 Jane M. Ussher, *Women and Madness, Myth and Experience* (London: Routledge, 2011), 1.

Upgraded and Updated: On Hormone Replacement and Alleviation

Even though the terminology of PMDD has been formulated more than twenty years ago, institutes and research in its regard remain succinct.[9] As a result, the production of knowledge and treatments are scarce, and often reductive. PMDD, being a disease with hormonal and psychological impacts, usually has two types of actions proposed to the patient: a) birth control, aiming to suppress hormonal fluctuations and their impact on the body and the mind or b) antidepressants, hopefully alleviating the mental burden of the condition in the patient's everyday life. Even though these treatments might help some individuals by lessening the symptoms generated by the condition, it does not change anything regarding the lack of knowledge—both 'treatments' act merely as symptom control.

9 National Institutes of Health, "Sex Hormone-Sensitive Gene Complex Linked to Premenstrual Mood," January 3, 2017.

Our bodies are stuffed with pills to cope with PMDD symptoms while the disease itself remains a mystery, a pain overlooked, even hidden. In *Fake Periods, Side Effects, and Other Things,* naturopath Lara Briden explains how the (limited) number of solutions given to menstruating bodies reflects the scope of knowledge around the topic. *'At the moment, the pill is one of the only women's health treatments available to doctors,'* Briden says. *'So, of course, they have no choice but to prescribe it for all manner of period problems.'*[10]

As a result of these rhetorical choices, these bodies and their technology are still dismissed, put aside rather than questioned and supported. What will happen to these conditions if they remain buried? Are they veiled by the designed cure, be it the pill, the painkiller, or another subliminal lie?

I, too, recall choosing and loving birth control. I remember being told that the perfect cycle's length is 28 days. Exactly the same as the number of hormonal contraception pills I had to swallow. Before I got on birth control, I used to notice how my behaviour changed around that time. The texture of my discharges. The smell of my body. The way I looked at men. Ovulation is the key moment in which one should conceive, to have a higher chance of reproduction. My body knows that by now, but this was not always the case.

Summer 2016: I get prescribed Diane 35, a rather strong contraception pill, to deal with skin problems and non-existent periods. I'm pretty sure my body is trying to tell me something, but I'm nineteen and don't have time to wait for my skin to be perfect and my cycle to regulate. These are problems for early teens or older people, not for me.

I remember walking in the streets of Sicily with my ex. He gets mad because men look at me as if I'm an object. Am I not, though? Diane 35 cleared my skin, made my boobs grow, my hair thicken. It's all I ever wanted, all of this potential in a ridiculously tiny, plastic package. I am youth and elasticity in a box, it stretches for all the world to see. Now, I can decide if I want to bleed or not, simply by taking pills every month. I am ready to be used. Consumed. Taken. Everyone around me can sense this. The utopia of my body and my relationship doesn't last very long: I soon realise that the pill cuts off my appetite, my desire, and my libido. Suddenly, I have become this desirable object that cannot be consumed. My ex and I seemed to exist in perfect disharmony: one body hooked on natural testosterone—something the male body naturally produces—another controlled by artificial oestrogen. Horrible how cliché this sounds, and how grounded it feels. In retrospect, our dysfunctionality has become clearer to me. Being on Diane 35 is akin to getting a free ticket to the buffet when you've just lost your appetite. A luxurious hotel without a swimming pool. A reminder that it's impossible to get everything in life.

10 Jody Scott, "Fake Periods, Side Effects, and Other Things You Need to Know about the Pill," *Vogue Australia*, 2018.

In *No One Has to Get Their Period Anymore*, journalist Marion Renault illustrates the dilemma that exists in a society where many menstruating bodies would rather *not* experience the biological bleeding of their body. Reasons for such choices are sometimes linked to intense or unbearable pain, body dysphoria, or the lack of access to products or resources for menstruation. Still, an underlying desire remains to function optimally–or, better yet, compete with other individuals who aren't menstruating simply because they cannot. In the article, Renault interviews Yen, a mother of two: *'I want them to be competitive against those who don't have uteruses. Teenage years are so turbulent and horrific as is. I don't want them to suffer unnecessarily—and I can alleviate this for my child.'*[11]

This thought has probably appeared in many of our minds. Given the conditions in which our bodies evolve, no one could say it's not a valid and thoroughly understandable idea. Who wouldn't think this in a society where the conditions related to our reproductive systems are barely studied, and paid leave due to these pains or disability are extremely rare? The newest efficiency dream is not to menstruate, and, therefore, not to have these conditions. It's an idyll because, in this situation, our body would not be limited by its biological conditions. A world where we could be functional and optimal, where our body would not be an obstacle to our various activities and ambitions. But who sold us this dream? Why should we be *optimal* at all, and for whom?

In these artificial attempts to cure and hide, nothing deeper is investigated. Coming back to the testimony of Briden, the naturopath unpacks how *'pill bleeds are pharmaceutically induced bleeds... to reassure you that your body is doing something natural.'*[12] She then goes on: *'Many doctors continue to prescribe birth control to "normalize periods" and "regulate hormones", as though the pill's steroids are somehow equal to, or better than, your own hormones. The fact is, nothing could be further than the truth. Pill steroids are not better than your hormones. They're not even real hormones.'*[13] Will we resolve these conditions and treatments by simply eradicating and replacing natural hormones? Is that all we know? When looking at birth control and its use for emancipation and transformation, we can observe how they simulate the real, the biological bleed, to convince the 'naturality' of their essence. As if our distinction with 'nature' and the choices of some individuals to alter their biology wasn't fully accepted yet.

Still, at the end of the day, what everyone wants is just to have a smooth, enjoyable ride. When 'naturalistic' and 'holistic' strategies don't seem to work, pain and suffering call out for other treatments. Frequently, people opt for pills, pain relievers, and other medications out of necessity, or because they have a proven track record of effectively alleviating pain. The second-most administered treatment offered to PMDD sufferers, antidepressants, appears to support the thesis regarding the psychological

11 Marion Renault, "No One Has to Get Their Period Anymore," *The Atlantic*, July 23, 2018.

12 Scott, "Fake Periods," 2018.

13 Scott, "Fake Periods," 2018.

consequences of the condition by showing positive results. While the body seems to react to the presence of oestrogen correctly, the main hormone induced within the first two weeks of each month, progesterone, which arrives right after ovulation, seems to be the culprit of sudden changes in mood, embodiment, and perception. Antidepressants aim to overcome the despair and depressive moments generated by this hormonal change, smoothing over the monthly journey. But even if those treatments can ease one's experience of their body, we should not forget to demand changes within society, so that those bodies do not feel so sick and oppressed in the first place.

In the aforementioned *Women and Madness*, Ussher expands her question to a broader range of conditions attributed to female and menstruating bodies: *'I thus turn my gaze onto three other manifestations of madness ascribed to significant proportions of the female population: borderline personality disorder (BPD), post-traumatic stress disorder (PTSD), and premenstrual dysphoric disorder (PMDD). While my arguments can be generalized to other "female maladies" (such as anorexia or anxiety disorders), these three psychiatric disorders are ideal examples of the pathologization of women's reasonable response to restricted and repressive lives.'*[14] By underlying the generalisation around such conditions and their labelling, Ussher invites us to wonder: how can we consider the social component of these psychological issues? Greater design of technologies and cures should not *hide* the external factors a patient deals with, but rather aim to redefine the context this patient exists in.

Although PMDD can indeed be hereditary, studies demonstrate a clear correlation between discrimination, poverty, pressure to assimilate, and the appearance of such a condition or its aggravation.[15] It would be tempting, albeit hypocritical, not to see a direct link between these conditions and the standards of our capitalist society. In between the cracks of our world's mechanisms, patriarchy and psychiatry. While PMS and PMDD are now universally known and understood as limiting and hurtful conditions, their metaphors haven't ceased to exist. In their daily life, menstruating bodies might still try their best to perform and hide physical or psychological pain as a way to counteract the cliché's and stigmas that accompany womanhood (and, often, its anger). They conceal their day-to-day experience in order not to be discriminated against. Not to be judged. While many fight for these conditions' visibility, another parallel battlefield exists, one that deals with the recognition of the incapacity to perform and live *optimally*.

In 2002, more than twenty years ago, Joan C. Chrisler and Paula Caplan published *How PMS Became a Cultural Phenomenon and a Psychiatric Disorder*. In this paper, both researchers investigate how and if social context influences PMS, and what kind of solutions are

14 Ussher, *Women and Madness*, 2011, 11.

15 Corey E. Pilver, "Exposure to American Culture is Associated with Premenstrual Dysphoric Disorder Among Ethnic Minority Women," *Journal of Affective Disorders* 130, 1-2 (2011).

given to those suffering from it. Their conclusion?
'It is certainly easier to take medication to restore serenity or create emotional detachment (an often reported effect of Prozac/Sarafem) than it is to take steps to make changes in one's life circumstances, and women are getting the message from advertising and other forms of media that taking medication is what they should do.'[16] Right. And here we are, twenty years later, with not much changed. Thankfully, an army of enraged bodies gathered throughout time to discuss and collect information that could not be found or mentioned previously. Together, they are reclaiming the meaning of 'knowledge'.

16 Joan C. Chrisler and Paula Caplan, "The Strange Case of Dr. Jekyll and Ms. Hyde: How PMS Became a Cultural Phenomenon and a Psychiatric Disorder," *Annual Review of Sex Research* 13 (2002).

FemTech, or In Between Holistic and Transhuman Perspectives

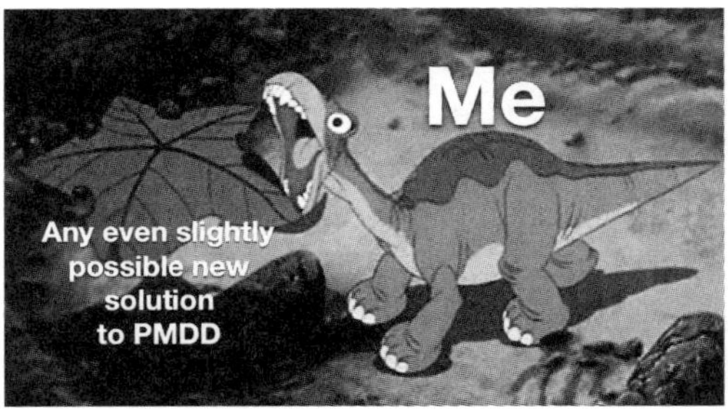

Figure 2 A meme posted by @pmddmemes on Instagram.

During 'hell week', the one right before the bleeding, I often feel the urgency to alter my body, or at least to change my perception. My detachment from people and physicality intensifies during those days. Human bodies seem bizarre to me. I'd like to smoke a joint, even though I don't usually crave weed. I bought truffles to micro-dose, but the prescribed amount isn't strong enough. When thoughts about past events pop up in my mind, these tiny balls of thoughts either explode into turmoil and anxiety or simply disappear in the overall fog that floats through my head. The perspective of some kind of relief feels far away, strengthening its urgency. It has become nearly impossible for me to write on these days. The feeling I initially wanted to start working with–*anger*–is long gone. Anger is the energy of beginners and amateurs. It's the fuel of those who want to throw out and hope to heal fast. Where's the line one draws in the sand, calling themselves properly sick? Why am I not choosing drugs? The pill, the SRRIs? No, not me. Who am I trying to be a warrior for? Shall I, as Preciado suggested, simply live in a world of 'molecular excitation'?

Whenever I felt most alone, alienated or misunderstood, I knew I could seek support online. The sense of isolation resulting from the lack of understanding has driven individuals with PMDD to seek alternative means of connection and support through the internet. Surprisingly enough, YouTube, TikTok, and Reddit have become sites for empirical testimonies ailing bodies can refer to. Within these platforms, one can discover poignant testimonials, heartfelt pleas for assistance, and inspiring success stories shared by patients who have found their ideal (medical) combinations to alleviate their symptoms. Once again, we witness the reappearance of the two aforementioned paths: one that leads towards comprehensive remedies and organic rhythms to heal, while the other ventures into the realm of biochemical influences, offering a pathway to freedom and liberation. While these ideologies share similar ideals, they differ somewhat. One aspires to slow down technological processes and their artificial changes, while the other supports the futuristic ideal of biological liberation through science and medicine. In a parallel manner, they both fundamentally question the standard design of our society.

While these online communities allow patients to collect and gather information, share knowledge, and support each other mentally, a new ideology emerged. A new and exponential market, one much bigger than the PMDD or PCOS market alone. One whose mission is to change the conditioning of female bodies, to vary the treatments, and expand its knowledge and accessibility: the world of FemTech. A revolution in the category of technology and digital health solutions designed to address women's health needs and well-being, including issues related to reproductive health, menstruation, and menopause. Now, how did this miracle come to life? As we started to face the deterministic realisation of our (conditioned) bodies, researchers and tech experts began to assemble. Together, they aimed to develop new tools and concepts to help our bodies and their technologies in everyday life. A brand-new industry born from the next generation of individuals, an army of strong, ambitious warriors ready to offer wellness, even a sense of conformity to menstruating bodies. Rather than adhering strictly to the dichotomy of *returning* to nature or emancipating *from* it, this new project aspires to carve out a space somewhere in between.

FemTech is an alliance of ancestral knowledge (or forms of rituals) mixed with digital devices and high-tech tools to enhance the experience of menstrual bodies. FemTech is a thermal ring you can put in your vagina to track your temperature. FemTech is a menstrual app that predicts the worst moment of your cycle to make a business deal—a.k.a. girl boss at her finest. FemTech is a DIY kit to test your fertility and its 'expiration date'. FemTech is your phone becoming your very own gynaecologist. Fluids are the issue; digital is the recipe. The world that Donna Haraway dreamt of mixed with the nuances of Silicon Valley. Yes. Finally. FemTech is what technology for menstruating bodies looks like in the 21st century. But what obstacles might one encounter when trying to design an advanced technology and newly invented philosophy for inclusion and care?

As mentioned before, an intuitive answer to this question would be to not only focus on fixing our bodies and ways to optimise pain, but also to think of objects and interfaces that offer care and understanding of our conditioning. Aware of such urgency, FemTech promises health and care to be designed by a more diverse body of thinkers, designers, and engineers. A groundbreaking idea, but a fragile one at that. One that needs, at all costs, not to gravitate towards efficiency or—God forbid—productivity. Such a revolution holds a huge potential, one that has been previously banned, eliminating the possibility to target not only symptoms but also the overall research, the gender gaps, as well as society's standards deeply rooted in patriarchy and capitalism. So, then. What exactly can science and technology do for our bodies? Which goals should we set? And, in the end, in whose interest does all of this happen?

We are, of course, not quite there yet. As this research field grows and grows, promising discoveries, self-diagnosis, and medication often seem to be the easiest way a patient can deal with PMDD. Nowadays, the internet still feels like a safer space to talk and investigate cures. While we wait for changes and dream of a speculative database where our bodies and conditions could be studied, even rendered real, society keeps evolving quickly, resulting in endless feelings of inadequacy—of not being optimal, not being 'productive'. Our quest for change and understanding isn't, however, just local. It is multiple, intertwined, omnipresent: a planet-wide call for care, for a transformation in medicine, a reminder to not just judge our bodily responses to the world, but also to question the world *itself*.

The Dream Girl

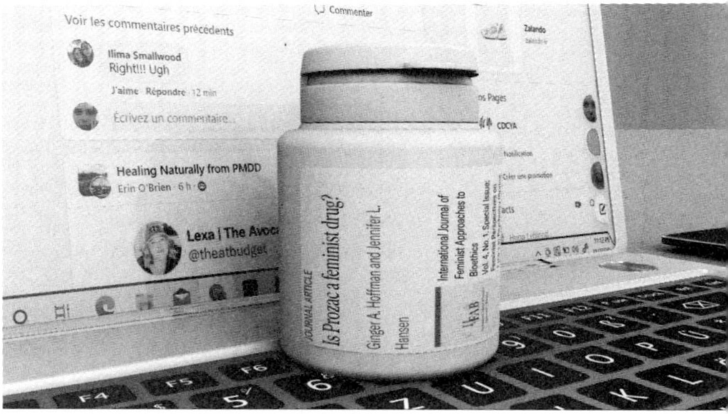

Figure 3 Rendered image, screenshot of the Jstor Library article 'Is Prozac a Feminist Drug?'.

I always love to shower around the seventh day: finally clean, finally renewed. Still not at my cutest. My hair kind of greasy from the hormones. In the evening, I grab my phone, and log in to Feeld. I don't know what exactly I'm looking for, but I NEED attention. I have a partner and great friends, but I DEMAND care. Something lingers in the way I carry myself, how I walk around the world. My stomach now flat, my cravings gone.

I am the dream girl. I feel hot and smart. I desire, and I am desired, I stare back because I am young flesh, young *blood,* and it feels so rare, so intense to feel adequate. Something in the smell of others, in their movement, suddenly I could hug the entire planet, perhaps even make out with it. Lips on soil on Earth on everything all at once. I wish I could be *that girl* all of the time, could live on a dazzling cocktail of oestrogen and serotonin, never get old, and always want to fuck. Twenty-four years old, in my follicular phase: I am now optimal, and it will never get any better than this. I wake up in the morning, acknowledging the time already passed, a time that will never return. I look at what I already possess. It's not much, but everyone says at least I have time; I have youth.

Youth is less when seen within the frame of fertility. I have been ovulating for over ten years, and still haven't procreated. Some rumours tell me I have approximately ten years left. Ten years left, as they say, to find the perfect partner, to 'get my act together', to carefully think and act, because this youth is only now, and I am a woman.

The memory of the fogginess from the luteal phase is already long gone. Forgotten. Forgiven. I can take the world back and chase whatever I had planned to do, but I have to remember: time is limited. Soon enough, something bigger, stronger, and wiser than me will again limit my thinking and actions. It's precisely because time is so short that I choose not to think of this evil, not anymore. Let me focus instead on what does work: the bleached locks in my hair, the hydration of my peachy skin. Happily, I notice the lubrication of my genitals, while I still can.

I have no hate, no. Nor do I feel repression: I go out like a trophy. I am above what is dictated, because I am exactly what I was intended to be. I will smile at strangers joyfully and perhaps fantasize, just for a second, that patriarchy feels like a distant battle, one I have momentarily won. For I am optimal. I could choose to love or hate, ride or die, date or break, but still, time is running out, and I should perhaps focus on what needs to be achieved, and succeed at it. While I still can.

Chapter II

The Internet is the Recipe: Sexual and Psychological Education in Digital Spheres

Perhaps the major complication we confront as feminists concerned about women, health, and healing seeking to intervene around the legitimacy of differences, is that this domain remains undertheorized and under-criticized while it becomes increasingly overmedicalized.
– Excerpt from *Revisioning Women, Health and Healing: Feminist, Cultural and Technoscience Perspectives* by Adele E. Clarke and Virginia Olesen

Sometimes, I remember how I tried to keep on behaving as if hormone changes and fluctuations weren't affecting me. The act of performing intimate or sexual relationships while I was bleeding, for example. How I feel terrible for the young woman I was then, who thought her sexual non-accessibility would cost her what she loved. Today, I would tell her that losing happens anyway, whether or not you impose certain matters onto your body. By now, I feel strong enough to accept this fact and let others know, but it doesn't suppress the discomfort of feeling inadequate, of not performing correctly. It's not just that I feel sleepy, disgusting, or that my body is cleansing, but also that I can't seem to be consumed or 'used'. Does this problem exist merely because of the world's physical needs—or at least, the people in it—as well as the monogamous nature of relationships? Or is it, fundamentally, a body-related problem that I myself should try to fix? Is it the format we decided to create, to seemingly protect ourselves, that oppresses me, or is it embedded within the nature of my physical flesh?

As I encounter the mirror, I notice new forehead wrinkles slowly appearing. The same ones as my dad. Those of ongoing surprises, or never-ending fears. By the look on my parent's faces, I can already tell I'll not be able to rock a wrinkle-free, baby-smooth skin for long. Too expressive, sensitive, and worried to escape the natural traces these sentiments leave on my skin. Twenty-four years old, supposedly at what people call 'the peak', but no strangers writing or chasing me anymore. Maybe they know, perhaps they *sense it*, they can smell the lack of sensual hormones, they somehow know, even before I knew myself, that I am not, currently, a fertile ground, and consequently will not consent often. For some, consuming flesh for the sake of personal storytelling, status quo and self-improvement, is a great recipe. I envy those, sometimes, but quickly come to terms with the thought that I cannot be one of them. Not today. There is something almost tragic, even romantic, about this incapacity to perform, this impossibility to be brave, to act. I cannot blame it on my partners anymore, but neither can I blame myself: it is simply the script that is rotten. A desire grows within me, to turn this experience into a practice of impossible quests. To be the wrong kind of lover, the lacking body, the non-accessible hole, the walking brain, the fearful, the un-brave. A desire to explore what can be found in this despair, thoughts that often find a space within the various gaps and holes of the internet.

Physically Limited, or Digitally Empowered?

As we've seen in our last chapter, long before health apps and FemTech devices even existed, the exchange of resources and information around menstrual and feminine care happened on the internet. YouTube, Reddit, and Facebook served as what I'd call a 'platform testimony' for those who couldn't find help through regular channels. Individuals who didn't feel understood or somehow weren't seen as 'normal' in their day-to-day environment probably recall sharing a post or a message somewhere, seeking help, advice or simply attention. Internet platforms existed as a receptacle, an open door where worries and conditions could fit, where they seemed solvable or at least softened through understanding. During all these years of posting and researching online, I do not recall a fear of being judged, or doubts about having my information collected. All of it was about support and community.

It is through this same digital platform, the internet itself, that I encountered the term *Premenstrual Dysphoric Disorder* for the first time, aimlessly typing symptoms and lists of burdens into my browser. There, I also encountered meme admin Chelsea, through her account @PMDD-memes on Instagram. As with many others, Chelsea's experiences and insights demonstrated the condition's lack of information and recognition. While chatting over Zoom, she shared how she started the account. Once she realised that there was not only zero information about this subject whatsoever, but also that no content could be found that made the topic less taboo—less 'dramatic'—she decided to create her platform. On it, she started to communicate about her relationship with the condition through memes and the use of irony.

Throughout our discussions, Chelsea told me the following: *'I had breast cancer last year. The first time I met my oncologist, I told her: "My cancer is a response to hormones; you should also know that I have PMDD."* She stopped, looked at me, and asked: *"PMDD? Premenstrual Dysphoric Disorder?"* I was so surprised that, for once, a doctor knew what it was. She put her notebook down and answered: *"I have been a cancer doctor for twenty-five years. I only know about this because my daughter has it, and she's been suicidal for the last couple of years. We had no idea what was going on. We finally found out that it's PMDD."* The doctor got emotional, and as I shared my experiences and the creation of my meme page with her, she said: *"I don't know anybody else who has this condition. I'm having such a hard time finding care for my daughter."'* This woman, an elite doctor, had now decided instead of talking about cancer, to try to get Chelsea's help: *'She was simply desperate to know how to help her daughter, who was struggling with PMDD. When you deal with cancer, such as breast cancer, which is affected by hormones, it's really important to understand these kinds of conditions, but she had never even heard of it before her daughter's diagnosis.'*

When I asked Chelsea which memes were generally performing the best, she answered: *'For sure, the ones relating to the unawareness of doctors on the subject, ha!'* This demonstrates how, on her Instagram page, medical misogyny and misunderstanding are turned into (wry) humour. As previously stated, exchanging thoughts on flesh-related issues, sexual lacks, and hormonal changes always seems smoother online. It is, unfortunately, a fact that when I was young, conversations with friends in which I could talk honestly about my body and my needs were rare. On the contrary, the internet and its digital spheres always felt like a safe space to share. In it exists a feeling of care and understanding I've never felt anywhere else. For a long time, I believed that the only type of acceptance available to me was a digital one. One that did not evoke the failure of my physical body. One that did not echo my incapacity to perform. In *Glitch Feminism*, Legacy Russell states how the internet embraces the failures of the flesh, symbolising the glitch as a representation of a fundamental error that doesn't try to conform: *'This non-performance is a glitch. This glitch is a form of refusal. Within glitch feminism, the glitch is celebrated as a vehicle of refusal, a strategy of non-performance. This glitch aims to make abstract again that which has been forced into an uncomfortable and ill-defined material: the body.'*[1] If this feeling of digital empowerment happens more regularly through the transformation of avatars and constructed-self, as Russel argues, I would add that this feeling of acceptance generally expands throughout digital spheres, and also plays a particular role in coming to terms with

1 Legacy Russell. *Glitch Feminism*. Verso Books, 2020.

self-acceptance and subsequent healing. While navigating those spheres, the improper and the non-optimal find themselves appreciated and valued for something that goes beyond their physical capabilities. Additionally, the ability to connect and create a community constructed around failure, incapacity, or lack, reinforces a feeling of belonging, one that gives strength to its agents. While Russel emphasizes the power of the digital sphere as a lens to observe the limitations imposed on physical bodies, it is valuable to rethink how the freedom experienced in those internet spheres could become an institutionalized and inclusive truth within larger society. To be digitally free, or cured, is one step toward validation and healing, but it should not remain the *only* type of activism our bodies can afford.

Facebook Group Rituals, or The Power of Collective Wisdom

Community is the killer app in health care.
– Steve Casey's speech in Revolution Health to the World Healthcare Innovation and Technology Congress

Sharing perceptions and testimonies online enables communities to realise one crucial thing: individual knowledge and embodied experience are highly relevant. Together, all of us can find ways to support, help, and gain agency for our conditions. If these online spheres and movements support bodies into feeling concerned for one another, or pro-active, they parallelly create a feeling of mistrust towards institutionalised health systems. In *The Healing Web,* researchers underlined how '*the perception of being supported [online] has a measurable effect on physical well-being*'.[2] Furthermore, they continue, the '*three most prevalent messages included participants' problems in communicating with their physicians, discussion about problems with hormone replacement therapy, and participants' identification and discussion of the advisability of alternative treatments.*'[3]

And still, for many conditions related to hormonal complications or, more broadly, to the reproductive system (PCOS, PMDD, Endometriosis), it is highly recommended,

2 Mary Jiang Bresnahan and Lisa Murray-Johnson, "The Healing Web," *Health Care for Women International* 23, no. 4 (June 1, 2002).

3 Bresnahan and Murray- Johnson, "The Healing Web," 2002.

if not mandatory, to be supervised and supported by doctors. There is no way to escape those encounters, and there should be no reason *not* to have them, seeing as these conditions, although not yet fully understood, are real diseases that deserve proper care.

Unfortunately, more often than not, these face-to-face meetings leave women and menstruating bodies feeling frustrated and misunderstood. *In Women Are Calling Out 'Medical Gaslighting'*, journalist Melinda Wenner states how *'research suggests that diagnostic errors occur in up to one out of every seven encounters between a doctor and patient, and that most of these mistakes are driven by the physician's lack of knowledge. Women are more likely to be misdiagnosed than men in a variety of situations.'* [4] Patients who feel that their symptoms are being dismissed as minor or mostly psychological are using the term 'medical gaslighting' to describe these experiences, and to share their stories on platforms such as Instagram. The internet, hosting various testimonials and experiences of those affected, sheds light on the insufficient acknowledgement and available treatments, thus exposing a deeply-rooted, pervasive medical misogyny, next to a severe lack of care upon addressing these concerns.

Beyond the topic of PMDD or reproductive health alone, recent years have illuminated the fundamental role healing, both on- and offline, holds within our current belief systems. The ideology of *heal thyself*, or a belief in self-sufficiency and auto-medication, helped many individuals regain agency towards their own life, choices, and conditions. Through both embodied experiences and scientific research, scholars have previously illustrated the significant role and relevance of online presence and support and its play in fostering a sense of comfort and adequacy, specifically for individuals facing unrecognised issues. To illustrate this phenomenon, which is not limited to mental or physical limitations, the article *From Lay Depression Narratives to Secular Ritual Healing* demonstrated how exchanges related to mental health struggles were actively participating in a positive evolution of one's mental state: *'The functional equivalent of the second step of ritual healing, the summoning of the transcendental is scured by the pragmatic forum dynamics, which evokes an authority in the form of the scientifically justified biomedical discourse.'* [5] Whether it was on Facebook, Reddit, Instagram, or YouTube, one could share concerns or survival strategies and hear them resonate. Indirectly, while those providing information lead the way towards a potential self-healing revolution, they also create social capital for the platforms, seeing as they provide data, connections, and networks.[6]

Naturally, patterns and similarities can be found within groups of individuals who struggle with similar issues; something made all the more prominent in digital conversations and encounters. Online platforms help these individuals: with a diagnosis, medication or simply a sense of *belonging*. But, of course, practices of sharing

4 Benjamin Bleicken et al., "Delayed Diagnosis of Adrenal Insufficiency is Common: A Cross-sectional Study in 216 Patients," *The American journal of the medical sciences vol. 339*, 6 (2010).

5 Domonkos Sik, "From Lay Depression Narratives to Secular Ritual Healing: An Online Ethnography of Mental Health Forums," Culture, *Medicine, and Psychiatry* 45, no. 4 (December 1, 2021).

6 Jessica S Ancker et al., "Peer-to-peer Communication, Cancer Prevention, and the Internet," *Journal of Health Communication* vol. 14 Suppl. 101, (2009).

and grouping together existed long before the internet. When one looks into the history of peer-to-peer knowledge in ancestral times, for example, many knowledge-sharing meetings between women organically occurred, often resulting in specific types of rituals. These encounters, feared by the Church or other institutions at the time, were quickly suppressed and hidden. Ironically, one could stipulate that the hegemonic platforms structures such as Facebook, Reddit, or Instagram supported the emergence of alternative forms of knowledge-sharing, subsequently facilitating these types of gatherings again. Through relational exchange and the public rendering of grass-root information, they indeed—to a certain extent—eased the connection between bodies and what they endure, offering a space for these rituals to be (re)born. While all of this allowed us menstruating bodies to feel more digitally empowered and mistrust the medical institutionalised field even more, it also brought to life a new alternative market, one of the never-ending possibilities regarding the cure for, again, infinite health-related conditions. But this process of constant search, coupled with an equally constant doubt, can sometimes become confusing. In *The Undying*, Anne Boyer retraces her battle with breast cancer, underlining how both institutionalised and personalised healthcare should be questioned. A reminder that through sickness and pain, all statements made by anyone involved are valid and yet aimless at the same time, and that finding a solution often remains a solitary quest:
'The pharmaceutical companies lie. The doctors lie. The sick lie. The healthy lie. The researchers lie. The Internet lies.'[7]

7 Anne Boyer. *The Undying: A Meditation on Modern Illness* (New York: MacMillan, 2019), 107.

The Growth of Alternative Medicine Proposals: Heal Thyself & Capitalism

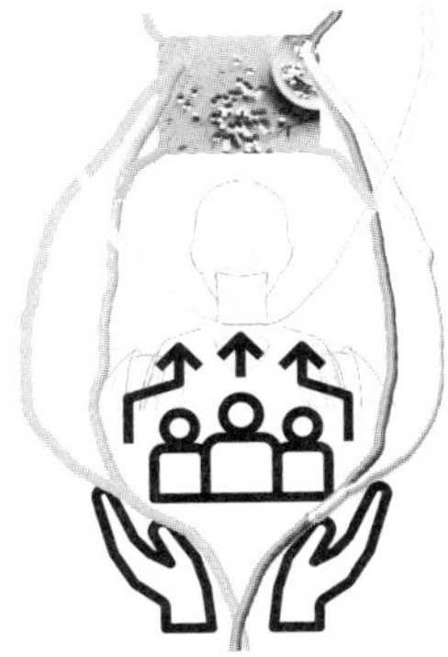

Figure 1 The internet is the recipe.

I take the Perfect Women's Multi. It has vitamins A, C, D, E, B, Biotin, and Folic Acid. Could I get these from a well-balanced diet? Probably! Is that a lot of work and planning? Sure is! Do these vitamins contain any of these vitamins? No idea!
– Excerpt from *No Ethical Vitamin Consumption Under Capitalism* by Arminda Downey-Mavromatis

As previously stated, theories of healing and self-medication have accumulated thanks to the internet and its networks. Next to this, however, the market for supplements and other recommended 'health products' appearing magically on someone's timeline boomed exponentially. These (online) businesses, of people buying pills and experimenting on themselves, give a platform to those who believe they know themselves better than others, those who wish to trial and error with their own bodies. Even though this might sound like freedom, one should nevertheless recognise the dangers and inherent elitism lying dormant here. Depending on the health condition, vitamins, gels, tools, and devices are offered to alleviate symptoms. Quite often, the expenses of these products (plus their shipping costs) reach a price level many individuals simply cannot afford. Although questioning contemporary medicine led to more beneficial changes and critical debate, the proposed alternative self-healing movement remains a relatively niche and, sadly, *privileged* option. Who can afford pills that cost you 50 dollars a month? And who even has *time* to do proper research to find these costly solutions?

I want to believe both the expansion of these supplement economies and the rise of alternative medicine came from a genuine place. A way to defy institutionalised forms of healing, almost a return to holistic cures. To baths of aromatic concoctions. To nightly rituals, and experimental diets. Numerous the options; diverse the practices. However, while these activities mostly happen without risks, inviting each individual to take responsibility for (the functioning of) *their* own body, it remains necessary to question these practices. How do they refocus the individual at the centre of their own health condition, making it, essentially, their problem? In *Holistic Health and the Critique of Western Medicine,* Janet McKee emphasises how *'these therapies also assign the major responsibility of health to the individual, lowering dependence on medical personnel, drugs, and other medical treatments.'*[8] More than a simple niche, this demand for alternative health treatments seems to revolutionise how we understand healthcare.

The Collaborative Care Model, an article published on functional medicine coaching, sees this tendency as a result of our current insufficient ways we heal and care for our bodies: *'With the rise of chronic diseases, long term pain, and more, the need for alternative healthcare practitioners and health coaches is growing now more than ever.'*[9] What's more, the research team of Brittany Eghaneyan tells us, *'patients are saying that the conventional model is not working, and they are now seeking and demanding an alternative option.'*[10]

Still, let's not forget: at the core of this alternative and holistic system resides an entire economy of self-taught practitioners and users constructing a whole business model of shipped supplements, plastic bottles, and daily vitamins. This ever-expanding economy, defined as the 'Complementary and Alternative Medicine Market', is estimated to be worth a whopping $404.7 billion by 2028.[11]

It should come as no surprise that all of these alternative remedies and holistic treatments are, to this day, barely acknowledged, let alone reimbursed. Additionally, their accessibility tends to differ according to each country's legislation or regulations. Luckily, many of these online treatments remain pretty DIY, a sort of 'ready-

8 Janet McKee, "Holistic Health and the Critique of Western Medicine," Social Science & *Medicine* 26, no. 8 (January 1, 1988): 775–84.

9 Brittany H. Eghaneyan et al., "Implementation of a Collaborative Care Model for the Treatment of Depression and Anxiety in a Community Health Center: Results From a Qualitative Case Study," Journal of *Multidisciplinary Healthcare* vol. 7 503-13. 4 Nov. 2014.

10 Eghaneyan, "Implementation of a Collaborative Care Model," 2014.

made' type of cure. Although access to this knowledge is public and therefore somehow accessible or free, one of the remaining differences when considering access is the time available for each body to experiment and the degree of possible danger if misused. This phenomenon also applies to many transgender individuals having to wait (way) too long for medication approval, therefore illegally consuming hormones or trying to employ alternative, holistic combinations as a replacement for the treatment they are asking for. By no means, though, do all of these stratagems replace the safe, fair, and equitable treatment our institutions should give each individual.

In the vast, sparkling ocean of internet recipes and DIY treatments, one should not overlook the many critical insights peer-to-peer communication and its various rituals hold. In the article *Peer-to-peer Communication, Cancer Prevention*, and the Internet, we can see how *'some unique and potentially problematic issues in online peer communication stem from data collection and aggregation. Even assuming that people post correct data about themselves (or correct explanatory information about health conditions), the self-selection of the participants reduces the generalizability of the information.'*[12]

It is seemingly not enough that all of this information, these resources, exist, that they are being shared, collected, and gathered every day, for they are still not recognised or legitimised in the eyes of science. What could be a proper model for this? Websites such as IamPMDD or PMDD memes pages relay information and play an active role as a supporting platform. They carry a clear message and bring awareness, even if they do this through questionable structures (Facebook, YouTube, Instagram) which can host and collect our experiences and our knowledge. Arguably enough, those platforms enable communities to connect, exchange, and share resources in places where the generic discourse does not tolerate any 'deviances'. But are they ever a *safe* space to rely on? What is being done with this shared knowledge, not only transformed but also *extracted*, after which it's used again to target the online user with precise online product recommendations?

11 Beth Ann Mayer, "Complementary and Alternative Medicine Is Becoming Less 'Alternative' – Here's Why," *Healthline*, May 19, 2021.

12 Ancker, "Peer-to-peer Communication," 2009, 38-46.

Capitalism, Product Recommendation, and Facebook Ads: The Platform Economy

Survey suggests it takes approximately a year and a half for a female to get bored with her sexual life or interactions with partners. I wonder how many partners I'll have to go through before I know this as a fundamental truth. For now, I exist in a world where I've been trained to think 'monosexuality' is the only way to keep my partner loyal. When I feel sensual and optimal, this idea sits well with me. But it never lasts long. Tonight, it's a full moon, and I'm ovulating. A stranger wants to go on a walk. It's four o'clock; we're sitting down in the Red Light District. Every bad decision starts like this. We kiss. I don't like *him*, but I like the idea that I'm taking risks, that I'm desirable, can do what I want, and it won't matter. The presence of an unknown hand on my waist, an unknown tongue in my mouth leaves me stirred up inside.

On that same date, I prayed and manifested an event for myself. Something will happen tonight. Sometimes, when I ask for things, and I end up getting them, I imagine myself blessed. Feeling heard and loved. I start to believe what happens is meant to be, and therefore do not question the consequences of my actions. A whole different situation it is, then, when I'm feeling inadequate and non-functioning: I blame my body, often asking for a sign of ableism. As if my flesh has to prove me right, instead of me trying to listen to it. From time to time, I am consumable. Utterly. This sudden sensual and optimal belief is, I know full well, not sustainable: only the full moon lets it happen. A one-day-a-month type of experience. I take this memory with me when I go to bed the next day. The knowledge of my sexualised body nestles itself cosily inside my brain. Curls up in there, like a warm snuggle. How many times did I wish for some kind of pill that could make this belief last longer?

Sometimes, I imagine this is what it feels like to exist in a constant flow of sensuality, with the right dose of hormones. If only I'd found the proper amount of supplements. If only I'd found the right recommendation online. If only I'd stuck to something *long enough*. I've dreamt about creating this *one* component, a tantalising, secret mixture, the one thing that could help me feel at ease, keep myself feeling alive from within. But alas. This emotional state, its ideal moment, never seems to remain constant, and I often desperately search for its edges, a place to cross. Often, this ideal of self-healing and empowerment through personal choices leads the individual not to question the support structure that failed them in the first place—instead, they get too caught up thinking, hey, I can and should fix myself, by myself. In *Health, Health Care, and Capitalism*, Colin Leys puts in perspective the focus of contemporary medicine, underlying how

'the health threats facing modern society had more to do with physiological and psychological abnormalities, broad and perhaps congenital tendencies to sickness surfacing among populations rendered dysfunctional and unproductive by poverty, ignorance, inequality, poor diet, and housing, unemployment, or overwork.'[13]

Unfortunately, the main ideology of healing within capitalism seeks to address issues only once they manifest—the typical symptom control—rather than proactively questioning the toxic, oppressive environment in which individuals and their conditions exist.

As we keep sharing our distress, our pain, or even our inability to function on the public display of online platforms, those platforms keep profiting from our despair.

13 Colin Leys, "Health, Health Care and Capitalism," *Socialist Register* 46 (2009): 1–28.

In these communities where one searches for comfort and help, the stream of pleading messages is littered with Facebook Ads, product recommendations, and affiliated marketing. Suddenly, this space for support and resources becomes an opportunity to sell: referencing products under the name of sponsors, making the theorisation of peer-to-peer recommendation even harder to test, qualify, and recognise. In *Digital Labour in the Platform Economy*, the business model of search platforms is shown to participate in the extraction of data and, therefore, to produce implicit labour done by the user. How, exactly?

'Compared to Uber, Deliveroo, and Foodora, Facebook represents a different ideal type, in which the labor performance is not immediately perceivable as a field of physical and intellectual efforts. Indeed, the digital labor on Facebook is the above relational activity, or "labor" of social reproduction.'[14]

Although it is by no means obvious to see these 'imperfect bodies' as exploited workers, they are nevertheless producing knowledge and effort through a platform that profits from them, without getting anything back. Ideally, we can imagine a world of shareable resources and internet exchanges where a peer-to-peer economy resembles a decentralised model. There, two individuals could interact, share, advise, buy, and sell goods and services directly with each other, without an intermediary third party, or the use of an incorporated entity.

14 Andrea Fumagalli, Stefano Lucarelli, Elena Musolino and Giulia Rocchi, "Digital Labour in the Platform Economy: The Case of Facebook," *Sustainability* 10, no. 6 (2018).

From Internet Resources to Digital Health Revolution: The Rise of a Female Health Agenda

If we can perceive the web as a fundamentally healing structure, then the walls of the virtual world should not become an ideal or referential environment. This approach simply needs to demand more from the medical institution and its structures: they should by no means get off scot-free. As previously stated, the ideology of self-healing and self-medication, often arising from mistrust and misinformation in the official channels, can have dangerous outcomes, ones neither the institutions nor the individuals themselves fully understand. Thankfully, more than just raising a community of self-educated helpers who see the possibility for real structural change and despise institutions, these networked connections reinforce both an ideological and technical revolution.

If, to look into the future for a moment, transhumanism keeps promising us its arrival and emancipation from our biological conditions, we must acknowledge that, for now, it simply isn't here yet. What's more, this project was already hard to believe in to begin with, given that science still doesn't *fully* understand what hormones are, or what they do to our bodies. Facing these realities, the ever-expanding gathering of individuals online leads us to more constructive and realistic observations: how can we send humans to the moon, but we still can't help certain bodies with their pain? The time for change has come. Who else but FemTech to take on a leading role in this?

Apps, podcasts, websites–multiple platforms show us this new ideology, FemTech. But this collective interest in women's health isn't *that* avant-garde per se. Looking at the past, the women's health movement of the 1960s and 1970s already transformed the doctor-patient relationship, which held the rather novel concept that women should take control of their health themselves (read: mostly male doctors didn't know how to handle it, and still don't). Through protests, DIY self-kits (such as those by the famous Del'Em) and various waves of 'rebellious' propaganda, women tried to ensure a new era of care that would go *beyond* institutional recognition and acceptance. Almost fifty years later, sadly, these goals still haven't been reached. However, it's hopeful to see a more global movement, one of conscious and physical awareness, leading women and menstruating bodies to develop a critical, caring attitude toward health and care.

With the technological and scientific fields advancing greatly in the first half of the 21st century, a real potential for change became evident. In the female health community, it was becoming clearer and clearer that their issues (battles for more recognition, mostly) were deeply rooted in society's mechanisms, whether it be capitalism, patriarchy, lobbies, or systemic oppression. We have thoroughly discussed this already. But, as a result, in the current digital health revolution, big players such as FemTech have many urgent discussions on their plate, and their promises can only be kept if their strategies are inclusive and diverse enough. As argued in *The Need for Feminist Intersectionality in Digital Health* by Caroline A. Figueroa and co, we can see not only the importance of including more diverse groups of individuals in the processes, but also the importance of including *'marginalized groups—eg, ethnic or racial minority women and low-income women into app design and testing and ensure groups will benefit in tangible ways from the research',* as well as *'increase (minority) women in digital health leadership positions and give them more recognition for their work.'*[15]

15 Caroline A. Figueroa, Tiffany Luo, Adrian Aguilera, and Courtney R Lyles, "The Need for Feminist Intersectionality in Digital Health," *The Lancet* vol. 3, issue 8 (August 2021).

If this revolution does not include these groups, it will be nearly impossible to attempt or even claim to make any difference.

With these challenges and obstacles, diversifying and revolutionising female health seems stunningly complex, perhaps even impossible to resolve. Countering this, the industry's perpetual updates, experiments, and transformations have unequivocally disproven such scepticism. Online, as much as in real life, there seems to be a strong will to change, hoping to mobilise the stagnant wheels of a decaying system once and for all. However, this contemporary 'digital health agenda' seems burdened with multiple missions and complex responsibilities running alongside each other. How to detangle all of these? The list includes establishing diverse, reliable public sources, recognising and revitalising past knowledge, and constructing trustworthy, secure frameworks for newly acquired testimonies. Above all, this revolution should not merely propose pills and treatments, but also healthy, alternative ways of living that discourage notions of competition, comparison, and relentless optimisation. We are not optimal. Nor will we ever *have* to be.

Chapter III

Elevated and Upgraded: The Paradigms of Female Health and Body Optimisation

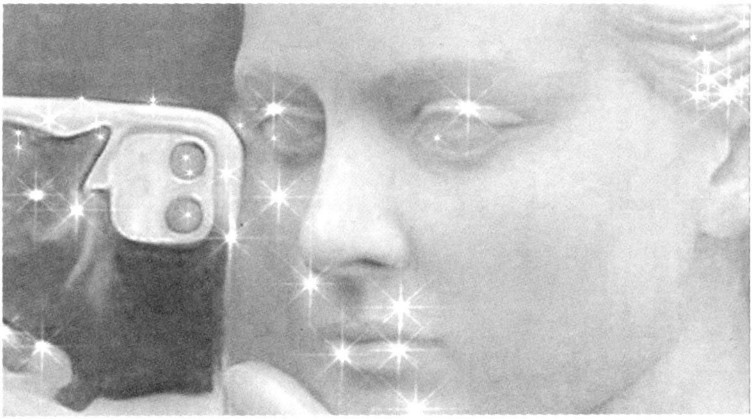

Figure 1 A wishful cyborg-goddess with glitters, by Morgane Billuart.

Optimisation

When I try to refocus on my body as a tool.
When I think of the best way to capitalize on it.
When I feel empowered because *used.*
When I know I am making the best out of the circumstances.
On TikTok, I heard someone say:
'Do you really want love, or are you just trying to find someone to survive capitalism with?' A quote somehow easily replaceable with many others:
'Do you really want to be perfect, or are you afraid to be replaced?'
'Do you really want to work so much, or are you too self-conscious to rest?'
'Do you really want to be THAT GIRL, or do you just feel like there is no other way?'
'Do you really want to be optimal, or are you simply trying to update?'

Evolving Not to Die: The Ultimate Body Optimisation

What if I told you that you had a tremendous power available to you? What if I told you that it would empower you to go beyond your everyday expectations, bring focus and logical reasoning, create better relationships, enhance your problem-solving ability, your creative insight, and blue-sky thinking, and finally, create deep insight and understanding?
— Excerpt from *The Optimized Woman* by Miranda Gray

In *The Optimized Woman*, Miranda Gray suggests strategies and tools to utilise the different moments of a menstruating body's cycle, hopefully making the best out of each situation.[1] If I read a text like that on a good day, I interpret it as an exercise—to see the glass half full—and as the only positive way to deal with physical challenges and institutional unrecognition. An optimistic attempt to make the best out of the worst while inhabiting a menstruating body. On a bad day, I go insane thinking about how our bodies are so well-trained to turn sadness and pain into

1 Miranda Gray, *The Optimized Woman* (London: John Hunt Publishing, 2009), 9.

profitability and creativity. Why? Why do we do this to ourselves? Realistically, one should not get mad at Miranda Gray, who's trying her best to make us feel more at ease in our bodies, trying desperately to empower us through the exercise of clarity, precision, and planning while we suffer through our monthly bleeding rituals. Perhaps this is the least we can do. Maximise a certain ease in our life, soothing our pain. Still, I cringe (and cry!) a little while thinking of this title, *The Optimal Woman*—when I think of myself who, like many others, trying to get ahead in a world that wasn't designed *by* any of us, *for* any of us. To be optimal, that deceiving trap of an idea. But what for? And for whom?

Planning your life based on your cycles is one of the many ways a menstruating body can become 'optimal'. It's about ensuring nothing important happens before and during the hell week. Quite often, this implies limiting your activities and decisions for approximately ten days a month. A rather big obstacle to our efficiency, to say the least. A practice that makes you wish you never had to stop, never had to pause, so you could endlessly just... thrive. Instead, you sit there, hating yourself because you assume your body is dysfunctional in some way, all the while putting in information about your cycle on the Clue app, and then you start wondering... *How great would it be if you could just cut out your lower organs altogether?* Could you then, perhaps, be optimal?

Some have compared a female-born body without hormones to a dried flower without any water. This is neither here nor there, and exactly the reason why post-menopausal bodies keep on ingesting pills. Around that age, while society and nature already dictated a sort of 'expiration date', artificial hormone intake can help you become slightly more functioning, remaining somehow 'optimal'. To either surgically remove the reproductive organs from your body or digest artificial hormones, all to overcome a burden—one of pain, one of idealised fertility—also means that the act of optimisation often resonates as gestures of integration, ingestion, and digestion. This doesn't just entail the processing of social constructs female bodies have to perform, but also the integration of external elements we need to survive. Oftentimes, even with these ideological exercises and integrations, our physical selves still do not excel in performance nor seamlessly assimilate into society. Even if these tools help us feel better, loved, taken care of, consumable, or 'functioning', they do not suppress the pain and despair that come with a quest for understanding. When Gray suggests a so-called *optimal woman*, she proposes a warrior, a body that is aware, educated, and privileged enough so that it can perform rituals of care in its everyday life. She refers to someone who perhaps has already understood the power beyond cycles, beyond patriarchy. Someone who could notice the impossibility of thriving consistently in society, therefore shifting obstacles into strength. This idea of a person, or more precisely, of a God-like woman, is a concept that has shaped and haunted us since the beginning of (wo) mankind. In many ways, to question the urge to optimise or to be ideal seems doomed to fail. Because, after all, who *doesn't* want to perform better?

In *Mythologies of Transhumanism*, philosopher Michael Hauskeller shows us in a brilliant way that '*to choose to be better is to be human.*'[2] Whatever the meaning of 'better' would be in his text, this thought underlines the depth of our desire to become a bigger, better, more advanced version of ourselves. This appetite for progress, profit, and efficiency is inevitable and, therefore, must be studied rather than eliminated. Still, as the philosopher argues in his book, it's true that '*the intention to create better futures for ourselves is pretty much the default position in Western societies today.*'[3] As Hauskeller suggests, when one thinks of body optimisation, it's challenging not to consider the concept of transhumanism alongside it. It is, furthermore, arduous not to imagine optimisation as a pure and simple '*sense for growth and amelioration*',[4] and even more challenging not to see this optimisation as a direct result of our drive for productivity within a capitalist, patriarchal system. When progress becomes the norm, our society provides less and less room for non-optimal and non-performative bodies, leading optimisation to become the ultimate Darwinian upgrade, rather than a purely personal choice.

Whether it comes to selecting a partner or a future potential employee, what stops us from always wanting to choose 'the better option', or the most 'fitting'? Who do we exclude when these criteria become so ingrained in our lives? Hauskeller insists that '*life is not a race, and ethicists should not have to suppose that it is. We don't necessarily compete with each other. [...] If the resources are limited, then we can only achieve equality by holding people back.*'[5] In our individual quest to become better, work faster, and produce more, an entire ecosystem hidden underneath society becomes polluted, often leaving behind individuals who couldn't even enter this competition in the first place. When we seek to adapt, we are told to do it quickly, leaving very little time to understand what we're doing exactly, or to care for—even cure—our bodies. Only a few privileged ones can afford the time to consider their pain, stress, or condition, and can do something about it. The rest of us are only able to hide it, curse it, or cover it up with supplements and medication to keep on living, to keep on hustling. Often, these ideologies are reinforced by books and sources referring to the ideal of a better life, a better self, and optimal health focused on changing personal habits. Once again, the burden of being perfect

2 Michael Hauskeller, *Mythologies of Transhumanism* (London: Palgrave Macmillan, 2016), 30.

3 Hauskeller, *Mythologies of Transhumanism*, 2016, 98.

4 Hauskeller, *Mythologies of Transhumanism*, 2016, 67.

5 Hauskeller, *Mythologies of Transhumanism*, 2016, 157.

falls on the individual. But, as previously demonstrated in this book, if a person's self-care and self-realisation are considered the initial steps towards establishing a solid groundwork for change, it's crucial not to disregard the structural pressure and oppression surrounding these.

Optimisation and its Genesis: An Ideal Shape by the Other

Boundless (adjective): unlimited or immense.
Synonyms: limitless, unbounded, untold, bottomless, immeasurable, measureless, incalculable, inestimable, abundant, abounding, great, inexhaustible.

What if we adults—you and I—could leap out of bed each morning and tackle the day with the extreme ferocity of an electrified tiger? What if our performance, fat loss, recovery, digestion, brain, sleep, hormones, and spirits were optimized and firing on all cylinders?
– Excerpt from *Boundless: Upgrading the Brain, Optimizing Your Body & Defying Ageing* by Ben Greenfield

Countless writings resemble this text by Ben Greenfield. In them, we can see similar exercises and rituals about becoming better and greater. No secret recipe, however, is disclosed–just a glimpse of extreme diets, supplements, and various advice towards a certain attitude in life. Optimisation isn't a process that only targets women and menstruating bodies: it speaks to everyone who aims to live a 'better' life, or even–why not?–challenge physics.

Still, when thinking of how menstruating bodies are dictated to live, how they're being portrayed and designed, the male gaze is a recurrent, if not omniscient, lens for, yet again, optimisation. When we pose the question, 'what does optimal look like when it comes to the female body?', it's a real challenge not to think of a girl boss winning, of *that girl*, the perfect girlfriend that never complains, the self-employed, impeccably dressed mom, the never-ageing, always pleasant, successful character of an 'ideal woman'. This ideal lives in our heads, rent-free, shaped by a culture of icons and designs—although these icons didn't necessarily subscribe to their role voluntarily. In *Body Perfect in a Capitalist World*, Azza El Masri underlines that in the 2010 movie *Killing Us Softly*, *'Jean Kilbourne demonstrates that technological advancements have been used in advertising to further engineer the woman's body to become an object of perfection.'*[6] During her lecture, as billboard images of never-ending beauty ideals and nuclear families pass by, Kilbourne states that a failure to achieve and resemble these icons is inevitable, emphasising how being an 'optimal' female body in a standardised, endlessly updated society is a battle lost forever.

The masculine desire to shape an ideal woman can be found in numerous stories and mythologies, tales told throughout the ages. Pygmalion, for example, or Aylmer in *The Birth-Mark* (a short story by Nathaniel Hawthorne), remind us of the endless loops in our patriarchal world and men's ultimate desire to create and curate a perfect creature. Yet wishing for perfection isn't just about physical features, as these stories remind us, but rather about the *possibility* of accessing and controlling these bodies. Pushing for perfection in someone else's body is often a will to change, design, and claim what doesn't belong to us. It's aiming for control, fluidity, and, last but not least, profit. It's all about shaping the ultimate tool, one that can subsequently be used, loved, and consumed. In these tales, male characters end up being punished by the gods for their attempt to shape the 'ideal woman', almost always losing precisely the thing they love. In real life, however, these male protagonists lose nothing: they survive, thrive, and execute their designs.

In Roman mythology, the deity Ops is represented and illustrated as the key holder of opportunity, wealth, fertility, and growth. Nowadays, her name still resonates in *opulent*, *optimal*, and *optimised.* Little can be found about Ops, but her Greek equivalent, Rhea, tells us more about her role and figure. In Greek myth, Rhea was the wife of Kronos (leader of the Titans) and Queen of Heaven. When Kronos heard he'd be deposed by one of his children, he decided to swallow every one of them as soon as they were born. Rhea took her youngest child, Zeus, and hid him

6 Azza El. Masri, "Body Perfect in a Capitalist World: An Analysis of Consumer Culture and the Perfect Body Image." Research paper, April 22, 2013.

away in a cave in Crete, saving him from being devoured. Instead, she presented Kronos with a stone wrapped in swaddling clothes, which he promptly ate. Scared of the survival of a—potentially—fitter son, Kronos decided to eat his own offspring, thus killing a progenitor born himself from the deity of fertility.

On the one hand, this story reminds us of fertility and body accessibility as primary symbols of opulence and optimality. Put into context: a body supplied with a womb will have its optimal standards connected to the capacity to give birth, to be accessed *as a womb.* On the other hand, though, Rhea's tale reminds us that, even though her body, with *her* womb, is hers to maintain—including its potential for profit and opulence—in the end, it's the *male* figure, Kronos, who decides which offspring should live or die. Kronos wants his wife to deliver this desired opulence, to be optimal, yet ultimately refuses the full optimisation process, which would mean him getting replaced by a younger, stronger god. Although this story was written more than two thousand years ago, Rhea's image and its symbols still resonate: look at what is expected of female bodies in terms of producing new life, how their flesh is being used, how masculine attitudes still decide on their rights, and their accessibility. These men, basing their choices on a deep-rooted fear of being replaced or dethroned, keep affecting lives, sometimes even destroying them.

When comparing myself to others, it can be challenging to recall who I aspire to compete with, and who I fear will replace me. I simply don't know anymore if this is about a gender dichotomy, peer-to-peer mirroring, or just societal pressure. After reading *Testo Junkie* by Paul B. Preciado, going through pages and pages of experiencing heat, hunger, energy, horniness, and constant anger, all generated by testosterone, my brain couldn't help but whisper: yes. This is optimal. This is how you can get anything you want. Nevertheless, the contemporary pressure to perform and be optimal goes beyond gender. While, traditionally, the ideal figure was often portrayed as an able, alpha male, in current times, this representation has evolved into something far greater than just *human* embodiment.

Optimisation, Bodies versus Machines

Figure 2 Optimal geo-scape quantifier with glitters by Morgane Billuart.

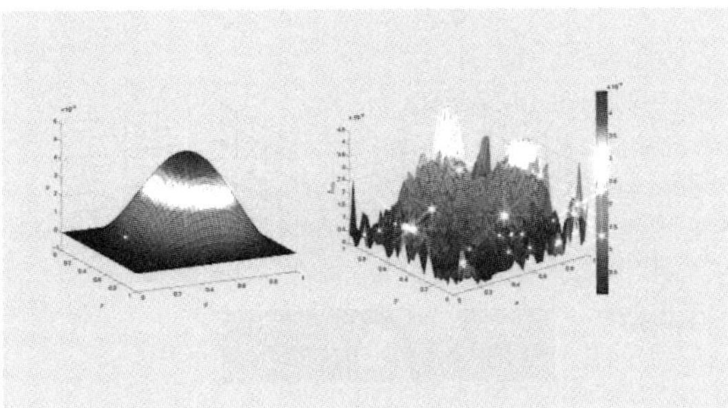

But, then again, nothing today ever de-escalates.
– 'Optimal-Self' by Jia Tolentino in *Trick Mirror*

Before seeking to update, to become the ultimate version of ourselves, one can wonder how the standards of capitalism, colonialism, and the endless longing for productivity have impacted this notion. Once, there existed a time when the word 'technology' was used as a synonym for progress, for the potential of automation. Back then, optimisation appeared as a concept freeing us from physical labour, by letting machines do our work more efficiently, more smoothly, and with less danger. Our workflows have never been faster than they are today, yet, as productivity thrives, our bodies and their labour have never been so pressurised. Machines did not relieve us of this pressure; instead, productivity spread its toxicity straight into our veins. If this need for optimisation can be seen within the context of company-building or profit-making, it's even more dangerous when discussing body performativity and idealised human productivity. Whether coming from an interpersonal situation or structures woven within our (capitalist) systems, there is no hiding from these pressures.

In *Mythologies of Transhumanism,* Michael Hauskeller reflects on the pressure within our psyche as well as outside of it, often leading us to think of ways to *cope* rather than finding strategies to *heal*, while being critical towards our environment. Hauskeller sees us being *'encouraged to enrich or replace our bodies with various bits of machinery, to use mood enhancers and other feel-good drugs, intelligence enhancers, drugs that increase alertness and our attention span, drugs that improve our memory, and others that help us forget, and even morality pills that will help us not to abuse any of those wonderful new abilities that modern technology has allowed us, or will soon allow us, to acquire.'*[7] While providing birth control for menstruating bodies with rare conditions, for example, or antidepressants for patients who are mentally ill, we see very little care given to these individuals to *reflect* on their unease. Moreover, this time scarcity leaves no room whatsoever for critical thought, or even for rest, leaving individuals with no other choice than just to swallow the pill, to enhance their existence with a quick fix, and think of the abundant ways in which they can potentially alter their everyday experiences—if they themselves put the work in.

7 Hauskeller, *Mythologies of Transhumanism*, 2016, 56.

Once we realise machines and technologies cannot help us live better lives, but instead have become the optimal reference for productivity, a new societal paradigm arrives: one of Promethean shame. In his book, *Sex and the Posthuman Condition*, again Hauskeller explains that *'Promethean shame is what we feel when we compare ourselves to the wonderful machines that we have created and realize how inferior we are.'*[8] Co-existing with this ideal of productivity leaves us bitter. We feel pushed towards an extreme condition, but still, we cannot rest, for machines have not entirely replaced us. *Yet.* In contrast, what has become ingrained in our minds and daily experiences is a constant pressure to maximise our potential, fuelled by the endless possibilities offered by modern technology. Sleeping less, eating more, endlessly doing, continuously thriving, watching the clock. As time passes, others are always doing a better job. The fear of being replaced, or even not chosen, becomes constant. Thus, the quest for profit is constantly expanding, never close enough to its finish, remaining a distant spot on the horizon forever. Although this pressure nowadays is usually imposed on both genders, it's relevant to note how the female body as an optimal, productive machine has a long history of visual representation: the fertile stay-at-home wife, the girl boss mom, and, later on, the subservient digital assistant, the robot sex doll... These female representations exist to feed a phantasmagoria,

8 Michael Hauskeller, *Sex and the Posthuman Condition* (London: Palgrave Macmillan, 2014), 114.

while also having a built-in design that prevents them from complaining about their condition. The representation of an ideal female as a digital asset, an always-ready-to-be-used product, was extracted from science fiction and placed squarely into our daily lives. She is Siri. She is Alexa. She is Samantha, Harmony, and Cortana. She is a neat little package of ready-made optimisation, without the nagging.

In 1984, Donna Haraway wrote in her *Cyborg Manifesto: 'I would rather be a cyborg than a goddess.'*[9] While it's likely many of us would also rather become Alexa than, say, Rhea or Ops, our options are unfortunately not endless. To refuse such an offer would imply refusing the benefits of progress, while also denying the natural processes of optimisation. In her manifesto, Haraway presents a perspective in which technologies support women in their gender emancipation and battle against society's oppression. Written more than thirty years ago, this avant-gardist, wholly optimistic perspective on technologies and their potential for humanity sadly seems to have aged poorly. Julia R. DeCook, then, dissects in her article *A [White] Cyborg's Manifesto* how Haraway's vision is not only limited to the Westernised vision of female embodiment and its forms of liberation, but also left us with a nostalgic idea of technology that was, unfortunately, never realised. *'Instead of shifting essentialized notions of gender and sex away from the body'*, DeCook tells us, *'the technological revolution of the late 20th and early 21st century may have further reified and cemented these differences rather than usurping them.'*[10] Many of these (female) cyborgs came into our lives, not to change things for the better, but with an intentional design: to be a better, more usable, more efficient female companion. For many, it's too alarmist to claim that these feminine tools and devices have become a *real* replacement for a daughter, a wife, or any form of companionship. What these examples help us see, however, is how the cyborg era failed to emancipate us from a binary perspective; instead, it just reinforced gender performativity, misogyny, and the notion of female accessibility.

Meanwhile, the real voices of human flesh who are, by default, less optimal, less compliant, perhaps less 'healthy', not as 'user-friendly', have disappeared into the background, a distant echo of tangible, imperfect life. Unfortunately, philosophical and theoretical perspectives on the questions surrounding optimisation are pretty scarce. Still, the few publicly accessible sources do not fail to underline their urgency. In *Optimization and Its Discontents*, researchers Fenwick McKelvey and Joshua Neves insist on reflecting on the social and political implications of such concepts. Specifically, they write how *'optimization [...] produces its share of discontents. In this context, it is tempting to think of various responses to, or ways of inhabiting, optimisation projects as forms of counter-optimization.'*[11] But, they continue, *'more than resistance, such everyday actions, habits of living, and forms of organization must be understood to be*

9 Donna Haraway, *A Cyborg Manifesto* (London: The Socialist Review, 1985), 65-108.

10 Julia DeCook, "A [White] Cyborg's Manifesto: The Overwhelmingly Western Ideology Driving Technofeminist Theory," Media, *Culture & Society* 43 (2020).

11 Fenwick McKelvey and Joshua Neves (eds.), "Introduction: Optimization and Its Discontents," Review of Communication 21, no. 2 (2021).

ordinary and constitutive.'[12] What, then, could a counter-optimisation look like for our bodies within the current, tirelessly optimising systems? How can we support individuals by giving them the time and affordances needed to live, rather than merely to *survive*? Instead of endlessly updating, what does our body need to truly heal?

When thinking of ways to recover from feelings of inadequacy, one must think about the weapons, the wounds, the attacks, and the oppressors beforehand. One must try to examine what shape the pain takes, and think of what exactly makes one feel weak, different, and–perhaps–improper. Sometimes, where these thoughts come from is clear: a feeling of inadequacy, a bunch of standards reminding you that you're not living up to them, figures that betray us, a sense of comfort suddenly taken away from us. Within society, it's both a miracle and a lie to pretend one can live and breathe in perfect alignment. No one, and we mean that literally, *no one* is perfect. Contrary to the machine, which is designed–and therefore closer to the gods–the human body, in itself, is imperfect, subject to changes, and, one could say, doomed to fail. In danger of becoming obsolete. Bodily experiences oscillate between waves of pain, pleasure, variation, expectation, and judgment–although that last one is probably just a toxic present from society. This human, bodily experience cannot, in essence, be completely fulfilling: it will always be lacking one thing or another.

I've often dreamt about being *that girl*, the perfect model, the exact formula others I loved seemed to project onto me. If it were up to me, I would have let them design me this way willingly, (re)shaping my core, claying my intentions, even programming my manners. Set everything into stone perfectly. If I could rewrite my own story, I'd wake up fertile, optimal, not just malleable but *consumable*, a smooth piece of hard candy sliding pleasantly on the tongue. I would have become *exactly* what they wished for, for it's within the space of fulfilled desires that love lasts and surely never dies. If one could only perform the perfect daughter, friend, and girlfriend, remaining this glowing object of desire for eternity. Imagine it, if you will. A fresh, young body–the most seductive image of them all, the figure forever praised; oh, what a pleasurable yet painful place to exist in. The moment one starts to grieve the idea of optimality, of performing perfectly, one starts seeing multiple illusions drift away with the tide, never to be seen again. All of these lies and constraints: the lie of consistency, the impossibility of eternity, the treacherous limits of the body. Whether in society's everyday experiences or interpersonal relationships, it's not difficult to recall the first time an external agent (a person, a construction, an expectation) left us feeling inadequate. Improper. Imperfect. Later on, obsessing over all those

12 McKelvey and Neves, "Optimization and Its Discontents," 2021.

who held judgment and hurt us, an eternal pain lingers, coupled with a profound realisation of our incapacity to perform. This lingering feeling becomes almost a moral value, an internalised criterium one applies to oneself. Oftentimes, these feelings of pain remain, sinking deeper and deeper into the layers of our skin, growing into an excuse for our miserable attitudes, our shapes, our lives.

In the end, I always ask:
Why do I miss the one that made me despise my own body?
The one that made me see the limits of my flesh.
The one that taught me I was imperfect.
The one that taught me about inadequacy.
The one that brought pain and hatred into my chest.
The path, once walked, that deception will walk
forevermore.

Chapter IV

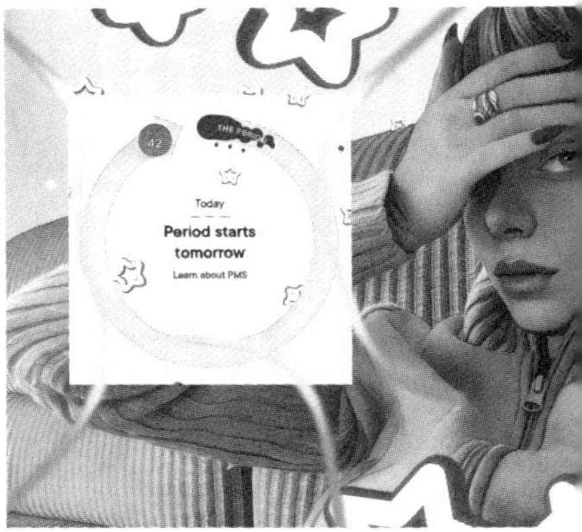

Gathering the Wounded Traces: From Self-Study to Data Collections

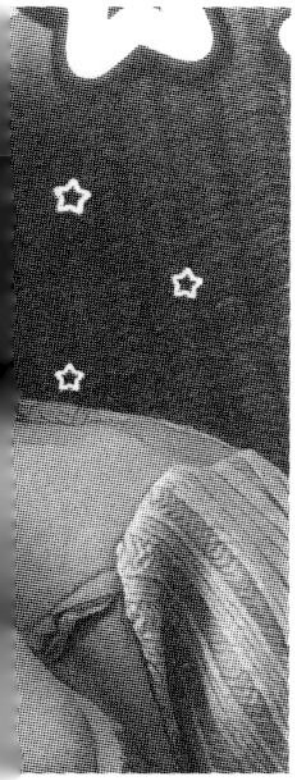

Figure 1 Screenshot from Clue App and no coping mechanism.

Yet another menstrual cycle that lasts more than forty days. The bitch isn't in a hurry to arrive, so my Clue app gently reminds me. Some might freak out, but I've learned with time not to fear pregnancy. Instead, I find myself contemplating the inherent capacity of my body to generate and regulate the hormones responsible for my menstruation, whenever it occurs. Before I installed any of these female health tracking apps—such as Clue—I relied solely on my senses, on vague memories of previous months. No other authority could justify my flows, their occasional absence. Self-study and self-acceptance were, for me, the only way to deal with my 'abnormal', 'non-functional' dispositions, all while dealing with unknown or poorly understood conditions—as we've seen in previous chapters. Like numerous others who encounter nontraditional fluctuations or menstrual conditions, I was astonished by the insufficient support and lack of knowledge within the medical realm. This enormous gap in knowledge and public information felt absurd, unjustified even. Searching for a solution within this vast ocean of bodies suffering from similar unrecognised, poorly studied conditions, I eventually realised I wasn't the only one noticing this. In our 21st century, despite all of the technology at our disposal, we seem to fail when it comes to recognising patterns and correlations, at least as far as the menstrual cycle is concerned.

As previously said, one would think that with all the data, information, and testimonies available online these days, the key to a cure is just one step away. For the sake of community building and healing, the current openness and flexibility out there seem without limits. While browsing online, an infinite array of Facebook groups and YouTube videos meets us, offering captivating insights, as well as reviews of unconventional products or experiments. Suffer from rosacea? This homemade cream with soybeans might help. Irregular menstrual cycles? Limit your milk intake; animal hormones mess with yours. Chronic bladder pain? Try steaming your body with these herbs, but avoid them if you have an IUD. Drowning in a sea of possibilities, cures, and homemade solutions, many scrollers regret that there isn't a platform to gather and analyse hard-earned discoveries. Where to capture all of these valuable solutions? Is there a beach where one can rest for a bit, cherishing one's treasures? As with any kind of treasure hunt, we know that others dream of this beachy spot as well. An interface to rest our weary heads and sleep. Suddenly, we are not alone in our aspirations: it doesn't take long for the GAFA giants (Google, Apple, Facebook, and Amazon) to embark on this venture with us. Once health data emerged as the latest prized possession, pharmaceutical industries and lobbyists swiftly joined the race.

Hey, you, PMDD-sufferer. Ready to give away all of your personal data for a potential cure?

When I'm at my worst, I'd gladly give up my privacy, all of it, just to give science and technology a chance to fix this, even if they're grasping at straws; anything to target the root cause of my issues. When it feels like I'm losing it and my peers are failing, too, I uncover a hidden agreement between us. An agreement to share and relay information as much as possible in the hopes of one day getting something in return. Screw intimacy; screw the illusion of anonymity. If we can give away something that contributes to a greater good, that leads to a better understanding of things, isn't that worth it? After all, sharing our feelings and symptoms on the internet enables us to connect, exchange, and *grow*. This ethereal structure holds us together. Why should we be scared to share even more?

When working towards a better understanding of marginalised bodies and disregarded conditions, one could think of a simple fix: collect information and produce books filled with the acquired knowledge, better known as data. Sure, the problem is structural, but if only we could look into the cause, not just the consequences, wouldn't we better understand our bodies, facilitate better tools, better cures? All it takes to get there is sharing our precious bits of data. So? What's keeping us? These visions of sacrificed privacy, even a loss of safety, have to be put into context, though: for the longest time, technologies and medical parties didn't have the best intentions regarding menstruating bodies. The most concrete example in 2022 is, of course, the overturn of Roe v. Wade by the U.S. Supreme Court, leading millions of womb-carrying individuals incapable of relying on their rights, unsure of safe, medical access to their own bodies. As this new law was enforced, the freely accessible menstruating apps and tools where one could share knowledge about their menstruating body suddenly became suspicious, *dangerous*. In an instant, sharing information with the digital world had taken a whole different turn, transforming a gesture of care and connection into the fear of being observed, surveilled, or even punished.[1]

At the start of my research, I, too, was naive enough to write proposals in which I aimed to 'simply' investigate the technologies (or workings) of menstruating bodies. Initially, it didn't seem overly complicated: the communities already existed, and were willing to share their insights and experiences. All that was left to do, supposedly, was to collect everything and (hopefully) render new insights. If we can send *men* to the *moon*, surely something can be done for our health and its representation in society? Well. It didn't take long for me to grasp the dark web of

1 Vittoria Eliott, "Fertility and Period Apps Can Be Weaponized in a Post-Roe World," *Wired*, 2022.

complexities sticking tightly to this endeavour. Nonetheless, every aspiration to achieve something must begin with a willingness to suspend disbelief temporarily. This here is my attempt.

Collecting and Archiving: A Small History of the Patient Equation

Gathering information, performing healing rituals, and exchanging knowledge about each other's bodies existed long before the internet was born. Secret meetings, as well as alternative ways of healing, were a big part of the strategies minorities, marginalised, disabled bodies, and women at large used to take care of their bodies when all other systems failed them. Through journaling, quantifying, and attentively observing their bodies and responses to various substances, these individuals expanded their understanding of the subject, subsequently enlightening others. They brought to the light what was seemingly beyond the grasp of science itself. As mentioned before, the history of these gatherings was systematically suppressed, resulting in a scarcity of resources on the subject. Fortunately, in recent years, interest in the practice of self-study and attention to our bodies has resurfaced. The movement of the quantified self, for example, underlines the need for self-awareness regarding our bodies and daily habits. Through rigorous analysis of one's day-to-day experience, quantified self movement invites individuals to collect and trace their bodies' behaviour, to better understand how it functions. With a minimalist design echoing the aesthetic of the care industry, the *Quantified Self* platform, a user-based website, presents its users with what appears to be common sense:

The Quantified Self is an international community of users and makers of self-tracking tools who share an interest in 'self-knowledge through numbers.' If you are tracking for any reason—to answer a health question, achieve a goal, explore an idea, or simply because you are curious—you can find help and support here.

– Excerpt from the *Quantified Self* website

Built in the name of 'personal science', this revolution seeks to alert people to their own agency in terms of health, care, and personal development. More than a simple journaling experience, its community investigates fundamental questions that feed multiple debates within the field of (digital) health. Similar to a cult–yes, you read that correctly–they embrace their practices, create tools and write books on the subject, while incorporating observations into their daily lives and diets. Simultaneously, Quantified Self members reflect on their own improvement, as well as the accessibility of their data and the design of wearables, sometimes raising critical questions regarding privacy and individual agency. At the heart of its design, this movement strives to integrate both quantitative and qualitative observations, a strategy long since overlooked in conventional medical practices.

Historically, tracking your health and other healing strategies were normative practices before they became a niche ideology on the internet–although they were never widely recognised. In *Measurement, Self-Tracking and The History of Science*, researcher Fenneke Sysling helps us contextualise how self-tracking is indeed rooted in the narratives of our world, and more specifically, in the history of medicine. From ancient methods of *'monitoring [our] body and its weight changes through food ingestion and discharges'*[2] to surveilling your diet and the smallest details of our lives, the quantified self approach has been embedded in our daily life for a long, *long* time. After all, isn't it common practice to try to limit our exposure to pain, disease, and discomfort? Still, Sysling suggests how this not-so-new ideology helped spread the ideology of contemporary

2 Fenneke Sysling, "Measurement, Self-Tracking and the History of Science: An Introduction," *History of Science*, 2019.

individual 'intelligence', while also reinforcing the *'increasing (self-) surveillance that our society requires and that this technology has pushed.'*[3] If the quantified self movement is a step forward in the race towards better digital health, it is not enough. Your personal diary cannot disclose what eating pumpkin seeds did to your menstrual cycle. Your iPhone's private notes cannot compute exactly what sleeping five hours a day for a week does to your libido.

On the contrary, apps and other digital platforms can be interconnected with many different parties who'd pay a fair price to understand the correlation between the two—libido and sleep—and develop a product fixing it all. Nowadays, as progress goes on, the quantified self movement aspires not just to collect and observe the body, but also to participate in the technological revolution of data collection and patient equations (comparing an individual's case with the norm). Books about such topics tend to have a rather utopian tone, resembling the failed utopia of *Gattaca*, the 1997 sci-fi movie directed by Andrew Niccol, starring Ethan Hawke and Uma Thurman. In it, optimality has become a quantifiable formula only a specific lifestyle can provide, and individuals failing to meet these requirements fall down the social ladder. Often, these stories depict a world where health is embedded in science, an inseparable merger, one where nothing can escape the control of data collection and quantified prevention.

In *The Patient Equation*, entrepreneur Glen de Vries underlines the endless change we could find if we could crack the secret of human health, somehow figuring out the best possible human equation. He tells us to *'imagine a world where as soon as something useful could be detected, be it a data point we can track with conventional medical measurements or a misbehaving molecule or behavioral pattern that we may not even fully appreciate today, we would be prompted to take action, use a medical device or drug, or change some aspect of how we live.'*[4]

Writings similar to *The Patient Equation* appear as a reference to better understand the ideology beyond such ambitious enterprises. Often written by doctors or scientists, these phantasms of a fully calculable, yet fearsome future are rooted within a debilitating observation of contemporary healthcare, and what it costs us. While observing the decay of a medical system failing to sustain itself, we see many researchers ask: what if we could cure and prevent people's diseases? What if our healthcare system was trained enough so that people wouldn't have to guess the cause of their diseases? The answer, if you ask numerous healthcare professionals, lies in keenly witnessing the decay of the medical realm as we know it, along with its inherent constraints of therapeutic approaches. So, basically: knowing what ails a patient before they themselves even know, and knowing without having to comfort these patients.

3 Sysling, "Measurement," 2019.

4 Glen de Vries and Jeremy Blachman, *The Patient Equation: The Precision Medicine Revolution in the Age of COVID-19 and Beyond*, (New York: Wiley, 2020), 12.

Aaron Fausz emphasises in *Healthcare Is Killing Us* the need to rethink a system where consumers are respected and in control, and where *'communities are focused on prevention and health instead of just on sick care and where pricing is no longer hidden.'*[5] However, as the medical industry slowly drowns in debt, becoming more and more privatised, the changes required don't seem to be happening, at least not without a clear sign of profit. More than just a new concept of health where listening and prevention are key factors, a book such as *The Patient Equation* shows us infinite possibilities for quantifiable systems, making us (hopefully) realise that simply taking the drugs prescribed isn't, perhaps, the most efficient. Fausz writes that *'so many things are so much better than drugs, things we are not even running studies on',*[6] which leaves us as readers to imagine a world where medicine could have a new meaning. One in which—can you imagine?—taking a pill is not the *only* solution. A world where cures exist outside of lobbies and pharmaceutical industries, a place that enables individuals to receive care without the need for forced system reliability. Sounds great, right? Alas, challenges in the medical realm are much more complex than the quantified self ideology alone covers. At its core, this ideology doesn't go much further than urging each individual to train themselves and get to know their own body better, thus getting a better grasp on their health. By analysing each aspect of one's life (the books you read, the number of steps you take daily), one could potentially crack the code of well-being, living a more authentic, transparent, and fulfilling life.

Unfortunately, it's impossible to think about self-tracking and performance optimisation outside the framework of our neoliberal system, where profits and exploitation rule. Whether it's to control, survey, or turn into a formula of product-based consumption, the economy of information and extraction wants you to heal, but wants to decide *how* you do this.

In *Quantified Self and Neoliberal Self-Government*, Thomas J. Catlaw and Billie Sandberg question neoliberalism's ambivalence in these new self-aware ideologies. As Catlaw and Sandberg explain, social groups often detach themselves from authority and so-called experts, reuniting with each other after several failures from the medical system to fulfil their needs.[7] Unfortunately, we can see that these 'outsider' knowledge exchanges are still hosted and shared on neoliberal platforms (such as social media, apps, etc.). In doing so, these social groups have moved from a structure that failed to support them towards a structure that doesn't necessarily want what's best for them either, specifically safety-wise, as is the case with various menstruating and health apps. Whether or not these platforms will distribute and share the user's information remains to be seen.

5 Aaron Fausz and W. Terry Howell, *Healthcare Is Killing Us: The Power of Disruptive Innovation to Create a System That Cares More and Costs Less*, (Nashville: Skye Solutions, 2019).

6 Fausz, *Healthcare Is Killing Us*, 2019.

7 Thomas J. Catlaw and Billie Sandberg, "The Quantified Self and the Evolution of Neoliberal Self-Government: An Exploratory Qualitative Study," *Administrative Theory & Praxis* 40, no. 1 (2018): 3-22.

Data Collection and Female Health: Self-Tracking and the Promise of Digital Health

Every woman is a self-tracker.
I wish I remembered where I read this sentence.
However, I don't.

This quote stayed with me intimately throughout my research; lingering in my brain, it told me that advancement in women's health could only truly happen if room was made for the experiences of these women or anyone with female reproductive organs. In 2020, I travelled to Coimbra, Portugal, to attend a robotics course from an engineering company that graciously welcomed a non-initiated student (and also artist). Of all the things that stayed with me on this travel, a thing called chronic cystitis (a.k.a. bladder pains) stuck out. Lost in a sea of numbers, math, and attempts at logic I hadn't encountered in some time, while also navigating Portugal in all of its brightness, my body was met with a constant, slight pain in the lower stomach. After various medical interventions and a confusing mixture of multiple prescriptions, I quickly realised that nobody (even myself) knew what exactly was going on, let alone how to treat it. Anti-bacterial medicine, antibiotics, probiotics, blood tests, urine tests... The list of treatments was endless, yet no trace of virus or bacteria was found. After several months of trial and error, enduring solitary and, frankly, distressing experimentation, and taking risks with drugs not officially recommended I had found online, I ultimately decided to return to France in search of better assistance.

This wasn't the first, and definitely won't be the last time I had to practice this sort of experimentation. Throughout the lived experiences of female bodies, it's rather intuitive to think of self-medication. A strategy no longer strange, considering the number of diseases misunderstood, unknown, under-researched, or just completely ignored. In Sexism Kills, Anastasia Lacina draws up an extensive history of women, pain, and hysteria, underlying the many historical moments that brought about medical misogyny. Sadly, she also emphasises how contemporary this matter still is. *'Medical misogyny'*, she tells us, *'has existed through-out human history, and it has harmed and killed millions, if not billions, of women. Does it still exist today? Of course.'*[8] She then hits us with the astonishing fact that *'of 2,400 surveyed female chronic pain patients, 90% of them reported feeling discriminated against because of their gender by their doctors.'*[9] That's only one in ten women who *don't* feel discriminated against at a doctor's appointment, supposedly a safe space. These haunting numbers of mistreatment and misdiagnosis are, of course, even worse for black or brown, non-binary, and trans people who, in addition to their pain, suffer from misunderstood, racist views of their bodies wherever they go. I am in awe when I see all these women and menstruating bodies fighting, functioning, and performing as best they can. The way these individuals move through many difficult daily tasks, both elegantly and silently, seems to confuse many people. Perhaps life is a breeze for them, after all? Various coping mechanisms blind those looking at it, thinking women (at large) are now at a status quo, and treatment is equal, that finally, our chances to exist and live are the same as everyone else's. What people tend to forget, however, is that if some individuals seem to be thriving, looking all shiny and optimal, they're most likely out of options other than swallowing their hurt in silence, painfully 'thriving' on and on.

Dr Gabriel Maté, renowned addiction expert, looks at the systemic questions of 'idealised' care by calling out, first and foremost, our oppressive environment. In his new

8 Anastasia Lacina, "Sexism Kills: Medical Misogyny and Ignorance of Female Bodies," *Fordham Political Review*, 2019.

9 Lacina, "Sexism Kills," 2019.

book, *The Myth of Normal*, Dr Maté dissects why chronic illness and bad health are on the rise. He digs into our concept of what is supposedly 'normal' next to different healing processes in a toxic society. With his findings, he uncovers a rather harsh reality: a diseased body has, within a healthcare system failing to empower individuals or address their well-being holistically, minimal opportunities to truly recover.[10] The FemTech movement emerged into the female health debate with a similar dynamic; that is, first knowing the cause of the pain and then—and only then—making space for healing. The primary goal of this revolution was, of course, to utilise technology together with healthcare to dive deeper into the understanding of our own bodies and overall health. By doing so, FemTech aims to address significant knowledge gaps around menstruating bodies. An attempt that, at least conceptually, echoes one of the greatest challenges of the 21st century. A concept that offers an array of solutions for a problem that, to this day, has not yet been solved. Still, mixing up years of rigid technological understanding and Silicon Valley designs with the fluid, ever-changing nature of individuals and their experience is much more complex. Surprisingly (or not), it's not at all easy to turn data of our daily life and emotional tribulations into ones and zeros, a world of binary thought and strict labels.

During the initial phase of my research, I enrolled in a data science course in collaboration with a company specialising in healthcare. There, I had the opportunity to meet Rob in 't Zand. After suffering a severe injury due to an accident, Rob scoured the internet for years, seeking support he couldn't find elsewhere. With a background in informatics and business management, he decided to start his very own project: *Health Thing*, a future social media platform dedicated solely to health issues. While exercises in the early stage of the start-up were mostly focused on the mental health of healthcare workers living in the Netherlands, the long-term goal was to connect more people through mutual care and knowledge. Rob kept on saying that the *Health Thing's* gamification would be the 'cherry on top', but first, we'd have to figure out a patient modelling formula and run analysis on dummy data to better understand the information at hand. And by *we*, he also meant me, for I had joined the team behind this start-up.

Mental health data collections and FemTech apps data input look much alike, as do their challenges: both rely on the user's willingness to share information about things that are, in essence, hard to qualify. Physical pain, brain fog, an overall sense of confusion, pain, the awareness of one's toxic environment... These two research fields seek to use both quantitative and qualitative data, thus hope-

10 Gabor Maté, M.D., *Trauma, Illness, and Healing in a Toxic Culture* (London: Ebury Publisher, 2022), 408.

fully rendering a realistic overview (and understanding) of a user's experiences. But anyone interested in these matters will quickly realise that human feelings, or bodily senses, are by no means self-evident categories. In *The Patient Equation*, Glen de Vries leaves us with unanswered questions regarding this quantification, instead inviting us to respect the *unquantifiable*. Still, this doesn't have to imply the end of all research on health and well-being, for this field has, by now, transformed into a real gold mine for both profit and potential product development. The unquantifiable notion of our daily experiences should not—and does not—scare the data science field and its true believers, and it is through barometers, scales, and numbers that one decides how the journey feels, how deep the love is, and how damning the premenstrual syndromes will end up being.

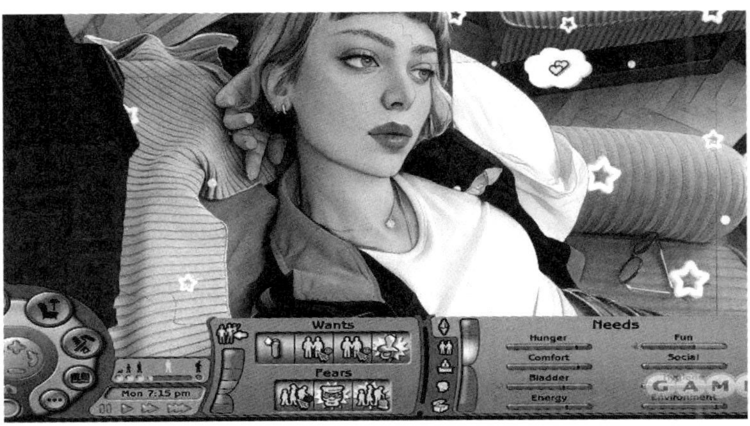

Figure 2 Screenshots of Sims' barometer score for happiness and well-being.

The Limited Understanding of Our Bodies: On Binaries and Data Feminism

Anyone willing to collect, label, and qualify life will benefit from using SQL, Excel, and Python. Once collected, the binary information arrives on these platforms ready to be treated, cleaned, and delegated with care. What does data look like, you might ask? Why, it has a goldlike quality, an air of complexity, is somehow very secretive and believes, perhaps, that its worth defines its design. This image of data might, however, just be how it presents itself to the outside world—with shiny shoes and a fancy coat on. More often than not, raw data consists simply of poorly inserted numbers or words from users who couldn't be bothered to fill in their information correctly. A data scientist's task, then, on any given day, is to formulate hypotheses about the collected information at hand, clean it, and then formulate a visualisation which hopefully confirms the initial hypothesis. While working for the *Health Thing* start-up, Rob's team and I quickly realised the difficulty of categorising data in such a project. How does one define 'satisfactory' mental health? What categorises as a 'good' life? What barometers can be used to assess people's quality of life accurately? In this haunting quest to better understand such limitations, I found myself once again surrounded by engineers. This time, no sunset above grand Portuguese hills was to be found, no lush parks on the horizon, but rather, loads of Zoom meetings with a nice little fake background of Rotterdam.

I feared this experience would be as traumatic as the previous one, but luckily, I realised quickly that I was surrounded by team members and mentors who were just as confused as I was. The beauty of men's audacity–having several of them on my team because, of course, engineers–is that they tend to ignore the complexity of the problem, not letting it stop them one bit. Onwards and upwards they go, not understanding much, yet fully convinced they will find a way. And so, throughout our mutual discoveries, we realised that it was not only rather complex to box these complex experiences into just 'good' or 'bad', but also that the use of barometers (scaled from one to ten) often limited the overall concept of mental health. To make matters even worse, our assumptions were challenging to formulate, and the data sets themselves were rather confusing. Some users were connecting to the platform multiple times a day to change their barometers, while others barely put information in about how they were feeling. Through the use of medians and other tricks meant to not let certain users' presence overtake our analysis, we quickly noticed how tricky collecting online information can be.

The aim of this kind of project–quantifying and analysing mental health to better cure or even prevent health problems–sounded like a fairly positive, worth-living experience. Unfortunately, the reality of its tasks felt limiting, reductive, and extremely tedious.[11] I do not (want to) wonder anymore why Clue is only giving me scraps of information about my cycle and its predictions. Getting additional analysis would probably cost way more and is, most likely, pretty much impossible at the moment, given the complexities of even the most basic analysis. I've said this before: the similarity between female and mental health issues and data science is that both rely on information that is essentially hard to grasp. Simultaneously, as we've seen within the quantified self movement, both rely on qualitative *and* quantitative information. Companies, start-

11 Vanessa Saba, "The Human Experience Will Not Be Quantified," *New York Times*, 2020.

ups or institutions overlooking these factors will surely fail to understand these phenomena, thus dismissing the exact thing which needs proving: a conclusion. Now, how can we render a more realistic experience of our bodies, one that is fully rounded? By using text, drawings, or the ability to choose more 'empirical options' on apps and platforms, all of which are valid attempts in the right direction.

Still, advancements in understanding our bodies through data suffer from many complications. In *Challenges for Big Data in Health Care*, researchers Clemens Scott Kruse and co underline the *'nine themes [that] emerged under the category of challenges'*,[12] which are, according to them, mainly problems regarding data standardisation and inaccuracies within data sets. Additionally, the researchers strongly emphasise how, based on biases and faulty calculations, the way data is collected to this day still replicates old systems of power, reminding us that the use of data collection is one option, but cannot be the only one. Furthermore, when looking at the quantification of human experience through the eyes of gender fluidity, it is clear that our current systems do not hold any space for non-binary people. Sidney Kung shows us in *Adapting Data Science for Non-Binary Inclusivity* how, for example, *'fruit can be either an apple or a pear, but not both at the same time. Although these multiclass models deal with more than two classifications, the aspect of binary categorisation remains.'*[13] Exactly this difficulty in implementing nuances into rigid data models and patient classification reminds us of the many, *many* changes still needed within the language of data science. If we want these tools to be able to give truly realistic, ground-breaking insights into the unknown, more attention towards the correct tools and proper selection of individuals is necessary.[14]

Similar observations were made by Catherine D'Ignazio and Lauren F. Klein, both data scientists, in their 2020 book *Data Feminism*. Their work, an in-depth analysis of power structures and requirements for fair treatment of users' information, is a must-read for anyone interested in these challenges. As they question systemic power structures, data visualisation, and the strategies of binary logic, both researchers insist on investigating emotions and embodiments, rather than just numbers. Most importantly, they underline how *what gets counted, counts*,[15] therefore, we must rethink binaries and hierarchies. If we truly want to better understand global phenomena, how can we make sure marginalised bodies will want to be part of the research? How can we ensure that they become users? How do we bring not only gender but also race and social diversity into it? For D'Ignazio and Klein, the conclusion is obvious: if we want to use data and design to change things for the better, we need to look at the most oppressed individuals first, and see how they suffer from systemic repression. Only through looking at these

12 Clemens Scott Kruse, Rishi Goswamy, Yesha Raval and Sarah Marawi. "Challenges and Opportunities of Big Data in Health Care: A Systematic Review," JMIR Medical Informatics 4, no. 4 (2016).

13 Sidney Kung, "Adapting Data Science for Non-Binary Inclusivity," Towards Data Science, 2020.

14 Kung, "Adapting Data Science," 2020.

15 Catherine D'Ignazio and Lauren F. Klein, *Data Feminism* (Cambridge: MIT Press, 2023), 97.

experiences of the oppressed, so they tell us, can we make sure their needs are covered.[16]

Let's go back for a moment to the idea of collecting information from social media or Facebook groups. Data analysis needs a lot of accuracy plus a lot of data points to construct a true opinion on human experiences. If we tried to extract those points from Facebook groups, for example, the quantity would surely be there, but what a mess it would be to classify and label each individual and their respective information! Haunting, to say the least. Also, not to forget: online information usually originates primarily from Westernised lifestyles and communities, making their shared experiences a majority of what can be found online. This doesn't mean, of course, that they should be regarded as such. If not only for the sake of inclusion, but also because it's been proven that medications and treatments have diverse implications, depending on both gender and race. To finish with a bang, D'Ignazio and Klein state: numbers don't speak for themselves. Consider context, please.[17]

For some, the urgency to seek help in a non-institutional way is pressing. They cannot wait for data science to become miraculously inclusive and caring. In *The Hologram*, activist Cassie Thornton proposes a system that doesn't rely on hospitals or specialists, but rather on a triangular group of exchange and care.[18] The premise of her practice is relatively simple: three people meet regularly to discuss how they feel, reflecting on the physical, mental, and social health of a fourth—the 'hologram'. In return, the fourth person participates in another group, where they are the care *giver* instead of the receiver, thus giving the system a chance to expand. A peer-to-peer network that uses the internet only if the connection is needed. A system that isn't dependent on vague promises of a digital utopia, but heals individuals right here, right now. This triangular care setup might sound like sci-fi to some ears, for we've all been trained—or indoctrinated?—to accept an individualistic healthcare approach as truth. But not to fear: activism and group organisation show us the power every one of us holds to truly change and support each other. If data science serves as an important gateway to explore these embodiments, these personal experiences of ours, then we must not overlook genuine care.

16 D'Ignazio and Klein, *Data Feminism*, 2023.

17 Kung, "Adapting Data Science," 2020.

18 Cassie Thornton, *The Hologram*, (Chicago: Pluto Press, 2020), 50.

Chapter V

FemTech: Discourse, Surveillance, and Privacy

Health services research exemplifies some of the greatest hopes and greatest fears for collecting and analyzing computerized personal health information.

– Excerpt from *Ethics, Law, And Aging* by Marshall B. Kapp

Aspiring to openly criticise technologies without offering ways to change them has never been my preferred modus operandi. Nor do I wish to simply reject digital platforms altogether or believe that every new form of digital creation is to be dismissed and suppressed. I, also, have no interest in becoming the sort of thinker that only focuses on what's going amiss without proposing any alternatives. Analysis and criticism should never be the end of a conversation, but rather the opening debate of what can be changed within a structure, and what it would take to do so. After analysing current knowledge (gaps) regarding female health, plus the critical, conceptual alternatives out there, we'll now focus more on a technical as well as critical analysis of FemTech apps (those who help you track your menstrual cycle and other female health issues) and their promise to support digital health. By bringing the complexity of these apps to the surface, I hope to bring along with it the urgency to rethink their design, thus avoiding systemic failures.

Flo, Natural Cycles, or Clue... All of these simple, digital calendars make one's body aware of itself, prepared for the storm that's about to come. Thanks to Clue, I could track, notice, and chase my mood swings or pains throughout the month. Certainly, I could have done all of this manually, writing everything I detected onto a calendar of my own, but I never did. If hand-written journals can get lost, and thoughts written on paper disappear over time, data traces on my phone follow me steadily wherever I go. In essence, many FemTech apps answer relatively simple queries: journaling experiences, tracing temperature, tracking fertility... The initial purpose of these apps is not to dictate the (desired) of a body, but rather to be able to observe patterns and unpredictability. For many, these apps are tangible evidence and validation of their experiences. Nothing else in the world could have demonstrated that, on my nineteenth birthday, I had gone without menstruating for a whopping seventy days. My Clue app did, however. Looking back, I don't recall my early time on menstruation apps very vividly. What I do remember is that in online communities, the names *Flo* and *Clue* were being spread around like holy water. Individuals started to check their menstruation tracker before actually agreeing to meet up. Planning holidays, work, long-distance relationship dates, all of this happened in light of the knowledge that, due to the menstrual cycle, one would become a monster for a few days, and one would have to schedule to survive, before slowly but surely preparing to feel fine again. All of this, I did myself—with the help of menstruation apps. However, my empirical research through these apps while being on birth control was, to say the least, biased. I mean, *girl*, why would you need to track anything? Hormonal birth control was planning these regular, pain-free cycles for me—so, definitely no seventy days without menstruating.

It was only a few years later, when I finally decided to go hormone-free, that I understood the full power and potential of these menstruation apps. During a constantly rushed, overstimulating daily life, one had the opportunity to sit down for a second and observe life's circularity. I never spent time searching through the app store, attempting to determine which app would be most suitable for me; instead, I relied on recommendations from my peers and decided to download Clue. To me, it always seemed like a relatively unbiased app, and in a way, it is: statistically speaking, it received way less backlash than Flo or Natural Cycles, which were either criticised for their monetisation strategy or the suspicion of questionable contraception forms as medically recognised. If the term 'FemTech' leads us to believe these technologies are here to represent a digital health revolution free of any concern, we should think twice, for a thorough examination of their design and functionality raises serious doubts. The current spotlight on FemTech has come at a pivotal moment: (mobile) applications are enabling the collection and analysis of data on various levels, therefore also facilitating the development of a digital health agenda and the intervention of devices in the most intimate parts of our lives. On the interfaces of FemTech apps, one can find 'visible', openly accessible data, such as close readings and content analysis of linguistic, textual, and visual data generated by developers or by users, as well as 'invisible' data, coded thoroughly into an application and accessible only through its backend. But what *are* FemTech apps exactly, and what kind of problems do they address? What does 'female health' mean through the eyes of the app landscape?

These past few years, health apps and digital health have been expanding continuously on app stores and digital devices, allowing users to track their mood, symptoms, progress, and overall well-being. As said in chapter four, within the context of FemTech, mobile apps are particularly interesting due to their unique, highly accessible distribution. Precisely because of their accessibility, as well as rapid circulation and affordances for user data, these FemTech apps have high potential to meet the promises of the field—such as legitimising unrecognised conditions and unacknowledged forms of pain—and to fill certain knowledge gaps.[1] Although its terminology might make its concept appear rather mysterious, in reality, FemTech manifests as a pregnancy test connected to your device, a menstruation tracker app, or a hot-flash journal. So, seemingly, nothing to worry about? FemTech and the broader agenda of digital health or the quantified self movement want to uncover notions and facts that have long been hidden from the public eye. To do so, they collect user-entered data, either inserted manually on the app by users or using small external sensors to detect things such as ovulation or basal body temperature. Later down the line, these apps process this information through advanced algorithms, finally arriving at a (hopefully concise) conclusion regarding the user's reproductive and sexual health. After a few years of using these apps, their usage feels mundane and completely normal, as if the app really knows you. Contemporary app landscapes, however, exhibit a high degree of platform dependency, plus often overlooked privacy concerns. With the two main app stores (the sites of distribution) owned by large platform corporations such as Apple or Google, the enterprise of app building exists within a gatekeeping paradigm, where apps allowed on the store are regulated through specific dependencies and models of monetisation. But what exactly are those apps? Who is their target audience, and what linguistic narratives surround their creation and usage?

1 News Desk, "Watch Now: Femtech Roundtable 2022 Can We Bridge the Gender Health Gap?," *FemTech World*, 2023.

Narratives in Female Health Apps

Apps that sell users a mediated, selective, and inaccurate notion of knowledge cloaked as a reliable form of self-knowledge, are critiqued as a heterosexist conceptualization of women's sexuality and problematized as an oppressive and overburdening notion of feminine self-optimization.

–Excerpt from *Tales of Self-Empowerment Through Digital Health Technologies: A Closer Look at 'FemTech'* by Tereza Hendl and Bianca Jansky

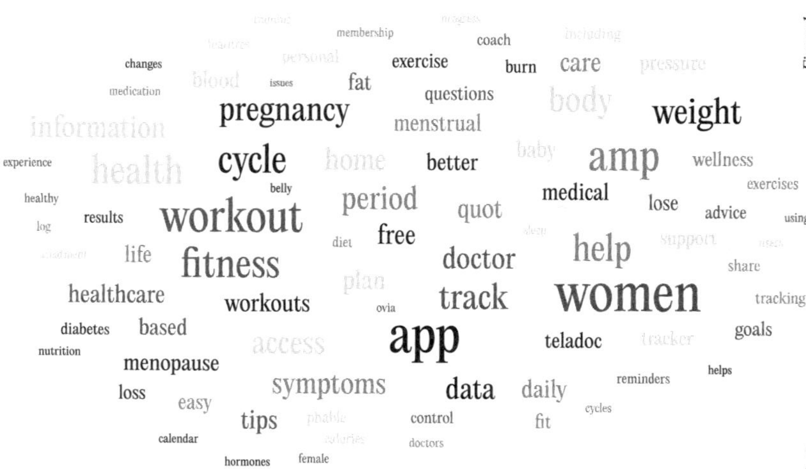

Figure 1 TagCloud for keywords in the studied query.

In order to gain deeper insight into the design and marketing strategies behind these FemTech platforms, our recently formed research group[2] embarked on a treacherous journey. To start working, we extracted the existing data of the 50 most downloaded 'Female Health' apps in the US. Flo clearly stood out as the biggest one in terms of downloads on the Google Play Store, boasting an impressive 80 million downloads. With this existing dataset, we set out to analyse several randomly chosen app descriptions by creating a tag cloud. In doing so, we tried to visually represent the prominence of specific keywords across all app descriptions, with the size of each keyword in the tag cloud indicating its predominance. What the cloud highlights (vividly) are keywords such as 'health', 'women', 'workout', and 'period'.

As shown in Figure 1, the first two keywords are close or identical to the original app query, which was, as previously mentioned, the one for 'Female Health' apps. Keywords such as 'period' and 'workout', though, hint at the type of thing that falls into the broader scope of 'Female Health' on the Google Play Store. Additional keywords fall into the same category as 'period', such as 'ovulation', 'pregnancy', 'cycle', or 'fertility'. The same goes for the keyword 'workout', with other entries such as 'weight', 'fitness', 'exercise', or 'coach'. It is clear, then, that two main domains stand out for our research purposes: we've got menstruation on the one hand, and physical self-development on the other. As a result of these rather particular narratives, many women and menstruating bodies feel left out of the discourse of these apps, specifically since they act as a reminder of their failure to ovulate, menstruate, or even experience regular flows—let alone hit the gym for some 'fitness'. In *Self-Tracking 'FemTech'*, Sara Roetman researched her own empirical experience with the Flo app, emphasising all the different ways in which the app commodified her experience into a slick, well-packaged design that somehow dictated her cycles, or even tried to steer them. She writes that *'when I log acne or weight gain, I immediately receive instructions on how to "fix my symptoms" from the app Flo. The app instructs me to do specific exercises, to eat vegetables, to change my sleeping schedule, and even to engage in sexual intercourse as "stress relief." The intimate and affective experiences of users are shaped and modulated by self-trackers to (re)produce and discipline the fertile and sexual female body to be both a productive labouring body and heterosexually attractive feminine subjectivity.'*[3]
As a result of these monolithic feelings experienced within the apps, many female researchers started to investigate just how these platforms reinforce hetero-patriarchal stereotypes, seeing how the aesthetics of such apps were not only soaked in conventionally 'sensual' and 'feminine' designs, but also that the discourse within and around these FemTech apps ended up falling back into a patriarchal,

2 Research done by Alette Schoon, Mathis Guerreiro, Morgane Billuart, Sne Scott Hansen and Tom Weber during the Digital Methods Winter School 2022 at the University of Amsterdam.

3 Sara Roetman, "Self-Tracking 'Femtech': Commodifying & Disciplining the Fertile Female Body," *AoIR Selected Papers of Internet Research* 2020, no. 21 (October 5, 2020).

consumerist approach. As researchers Anastasia Siapka and Elisabetta Biasin write in their research *Bleeding Data*: *'broadly put, the management of one's menstruation is conducive to better, more reliable execution of one's work responsibilities.'*[4] When one starts thinking of an ideal design, they add furthermore, or even a non-oppressive, gentle platform, things start to get tricky. How can this be?

Often, I find myself wondering what exactly it is I truly seek from a menstrual cycle app. What would be a good, neutral, comforting discourse on these platforms, for me and others? What kind of things do I expect when in need–is this support, acknowledgement, or product recommendations? A reminder that *no*, today is indeed not a good day to get hit by a car, no matter my mood? Every user's situation is different. Every menstruation app is, also. My experience of Clue contrasts with my opinion of Flo, as Clue doesn't give me product recommendations or targeted ads, and doesn't try to sell me stuff. Yet in a subtle way, Clue leaves me alone, also, lonely with my irregular tracker, incapable of knowing what exactly went wrong this month, or how I could ease my pain. For sure, there have been moments when I desired more guidance, information–some kind of input from these apps. However, the commercial recommendations that often accompany it are a tricky subject. For in the workings of these apps lies an interesting dissonance: when assistance is absent, the user feels its lack and is left wanting, yet when the technology is too pushy, a user quickly feels oppressed. As Sara Toeman's argues in *Self-Tracking 'FemTech'*, specific guidelines and recommendations from apps are also not at all welcomed by the user, who is left feeling like something is wrong with their body, endlessly wondering what they have done 'wrong', what might have led to their mental and physical pain. The question, however, remains: *why* and *how* do these platforms collect and analyse data, knowing that the result often is messages or notifications that seem excessively simplistic, almost reductionist?

In the article, *Health App Broke Its Privacy Promises*, journalist Lesley Fair investigates how Flo was taken to court for selling information to third parties, later turning these pieces of data into targeted production recommendations. *'For example'*, Fair writes, *'if an app user entered pregnancy-related information, Flo Health disclosed App Events with the word "pregnancy" in the title to the analytics divisions of those third parties. According to the complaint, Flo Health's disclosures of sensitive information about users' pregnancies or periods broke its privacy assurances to consumers and violated several of the third parties' own terms of service – terms Flo Health had agreed to.'*[5]
Rather interesting is how these articles are increasingly more and more difficult to find; instead, one sees loads of 'promises' saying Flo made specific changes and is now implementing a complete 'transparency' policy and privacy within the app. Right after the Roe turn-over

4 Anastasia Siapka and Elisabetta Biasin, "Bleeding Data: The Case of Fertility and Menstruation Tracking Apps," Internet Policy Review 10, no. 4 (2021).

5 Lesley Fair, "Health App Broke Its Privacy Promises by Disclosing Intimate Details About Users," Federal Trade Comission, January 13, 2021.

happened, Flo also started to develop a new feature called 'anonymous mode', allowing users to remove their name, email address, and technical identifiers from their profile. Nowadays, the search 'Flo+targeted ads' doesn't really get you anywhere, and traces of these past accusations are not readily accessible to the public. Considering the potential FemTech apps offer, it would be unreasonable not to leverage the available data to create optimal value and generate innovative insights. The way this is done at the moment, however, within existing models of data extraction and distribution, produces significant concerns. To make sense of the monolithic narratives within these apps' discourses, what might help us shine a light on their subliminal messages and design is the study of their categorisation, as well as their dependencies.

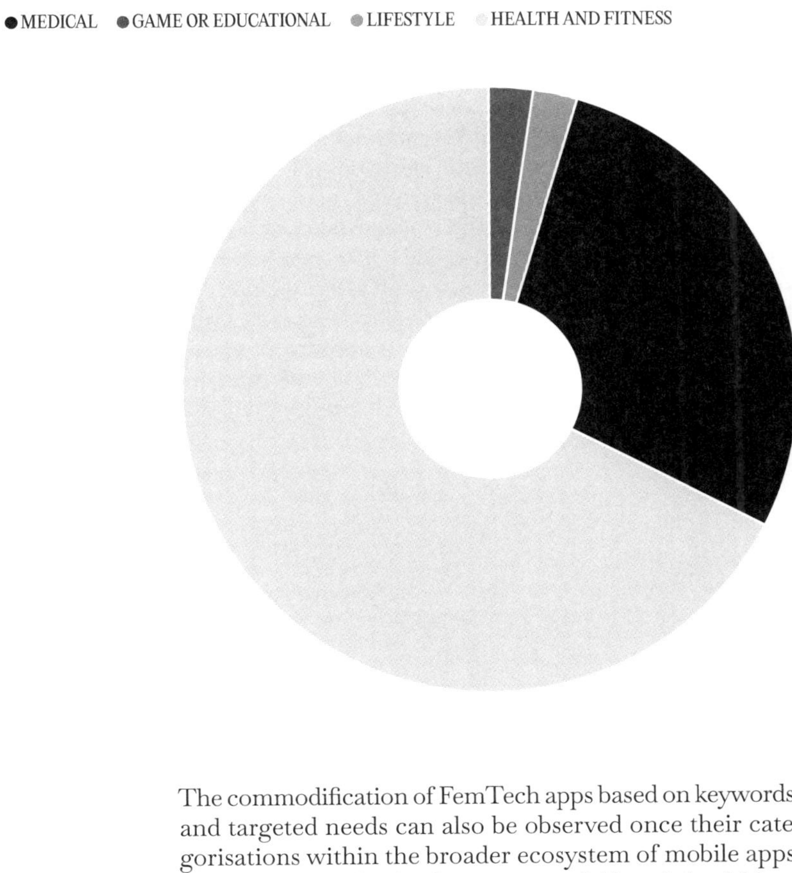

Figure 2 Apps represented by categories.

The commodification of FemTech apps based on keywords and targeted needs can also be observed once their categorisations within the broader ecosystem of mobile apps are analysed. Indeed, when you search 'female health' on the US's Google Play Store, as the above diagram shows, 36 out of 50 apps are categorised in *Health* and *Fitness*, corresponding to 72 per cent of the total sample size. As the graph demonstrates, the second major category of

FemTech apps is classified as 'medical'. If these apps are not exclusively found within the 'medical' category, one could posit that this is because they are not fully recognised or classified as 'medical' devices, potentially due to legal considerations. But what are the implications of putting apps millions of females use to track their health into categories labelled or understood as 'fitness and wellness'? In their article *Fertility Apps*, the New Caste Press Office introduces the research of Dr. Maryam Mehrnezhad and Dr. Teresa Almeida from the Department of Informatics, who investigated privacy risks that can originate from the mismanagement, misuse, and misappropriation of intimate data: *'Study shows that the majority of these fertility apps are classified as "Health & Fitness", a few as "Medical", and one as "Communication"'.* Building further upon this, the authors argue that *'miscategorising an insecure app that contains medical records as "Health & Fitness" would enable the developers to avoid the potential consequences, for example, of remaining in the app market without drawing significant attention to it. This means that fertility app data could continue to be sold to third parties for a variety of unauthorised uses, such as advertising and app development.'*[6] Of course, as expected: it often comes down to selling our intimate data. The categorisation of these FemTech apps also emerges as a more nuanced phenomenon. Not only does the fragmentation of female health into rigid, stereotypical categories lead to limited views, but it also causes regulatory (and even legal) challenges. As suggested in Mehrnezhad and Almeida's article, apps supposedly collecting 'sensitive data' but categorised as 'fitness' and 'wellness' are less likely to be held responsible or checked for privacy and legal accountability. So, how does an absence of clarity in categorisation contribute, then, to the pursuit of (female) body enhancement? And how is accountability for collected data skillfully evaded?

6 Maryam Mehrnezhad and Teresa Almeida, "Caring for Intimate Data in Fertility Technologies," CHI Conference on Human Factors in Computing Systems (CHI '21), May 8–13, 2021.

Privacy and Surveillance: The Downside of Online Care

Technologies do not possess inherent value. Their value is created by a business model that can link the technology to customers and monetize the results.
– Excerpt from *Business Models and Technological Innovation* by Charles Baden-Fuller and Stefan Haefliger

In November 2022, I met Carmen Hines, a young researcher and curator in Vienna. She was presenting her participation in the book Data After Nature, reading an extract of her current research on FemTech. Thrilled about another peer's research, I kept repeating the word 'FemTech' all night, and perhaps did so too close to my phone's microphone. As Hines started to read excerpts from her books, suddenly, a notification popped up on my phone: *Academia.edu: FemTech and Commodification of the Body — Still interested in this article?* Occasionally, I'll indulge in the whimsical notion that my phone can listen to my thoughts or some other uncanny way to know what I, deep down, really want. But usually, this is just me being silly. In truth, I've never been particularly concerned about the sensation of being heard, as—previously, that is—I failed to grasp the immediate implications of such data collection. I have nothing to hide, no one to run from, so I've always thought it is relatively harmless to be surveilled. My opinion has surely changed throughout this research, however, seeing certain countries' current political and reproductive climate. I've come to terms with the fact that I may have nothing to hide, nor fear, due to my many privileges: access to relatively cheap health care, a light skin colour, adequate knowledge about my body type, but, also, simply the privilege to live in a country where abortion is a *right* and not a punishment. My phone may still be listening, but at least now I count my blessings.

Back to the apps, then. How exactly do they deal with privacy and surveillance? It is, sadly, somewhat complicated and even tedious to determine precisely what happens to a user's data once entered into FemTech apps. Our research group, the one from the Digital Winter School, decided to check the possibilities Digital Methods offered us; that is, an insight into third parties and app permissions. (To clarify: a third-party application is an application from a vendor other than the device or operating system (OS) manufacturer upon which the apps are used.) Third-party applications can be either standalone apps or plug-ins that enhance the functionality of existing apps. Acknowledging these within the app ecology helps us understand the correlation between our FemTech apps and their dependency on other platforms. This dependency, for example, frequently leads to the transfer of information between several platforms, leaving users uncertain about where their data actually ends up, or what sort of privacy they have.

Firstly, let's look at *why* these apps even need third-party applications. (Hint: it has to do with an efficient use of time and money.) Third parties often accelerate an app's development, leading it to hit the market as soon as possible. Secondly, third parties are known to easily integrate into other apps, making it easier for developers to finish a smooth-functioning app in less time. Finally, the maintenance of third-party apps is also optimised as it is solely the provider's job to update it and ensure it runs smoothly, making it easy and tempting for app developers to use them worry-free. If someone wants to start building an app, it would be foolish not to use third-party services. However, their implementation is not without consequences...

During our winter school research, as depicted in Figure 3, our team discovered that many apps within our sample showed inherent links with third-party trackers. The bigger the bar chart, the more omnipresent the third-party

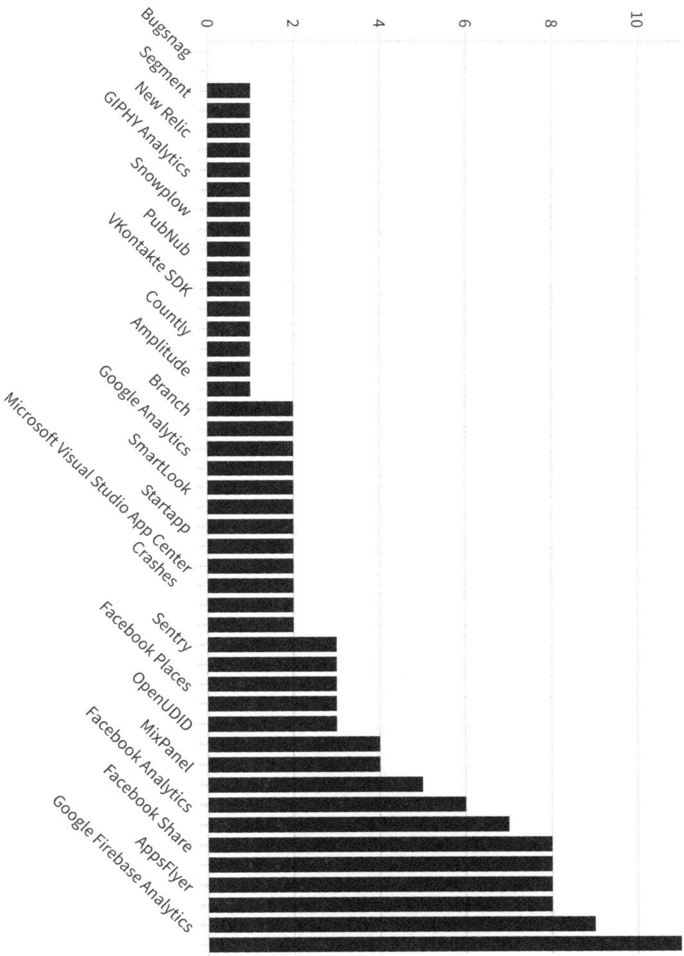

Figure 3 Apps and their third-party trackers.

tracker is throughout the sampled apps. As this figure shows, Google Firebase Analytics is the most present one among 'Female Health' apps on the Google Play Store, followed by Facebook Share, Facebook Login, Facebook Analytics, Google AdMob, and Google Analytics.

Clearly, the most common tracking services for our researched applications are closely related to Google and Facebook (*oh, hi, Mark!*). This, of course, shows a plausible correlation between our apps and recommendations generated by big data-player Facebook. It's pretty easy to understand why apps would want to share information with third parties: they gain said time for their app design and agency in shaping their users, providing them with more resources and recommendations. Now that we fully recognise all the third parties involved in the ecosystems of an app, it's even more crucial to examine the (sometimes grave) alterations of default permissions given by users in

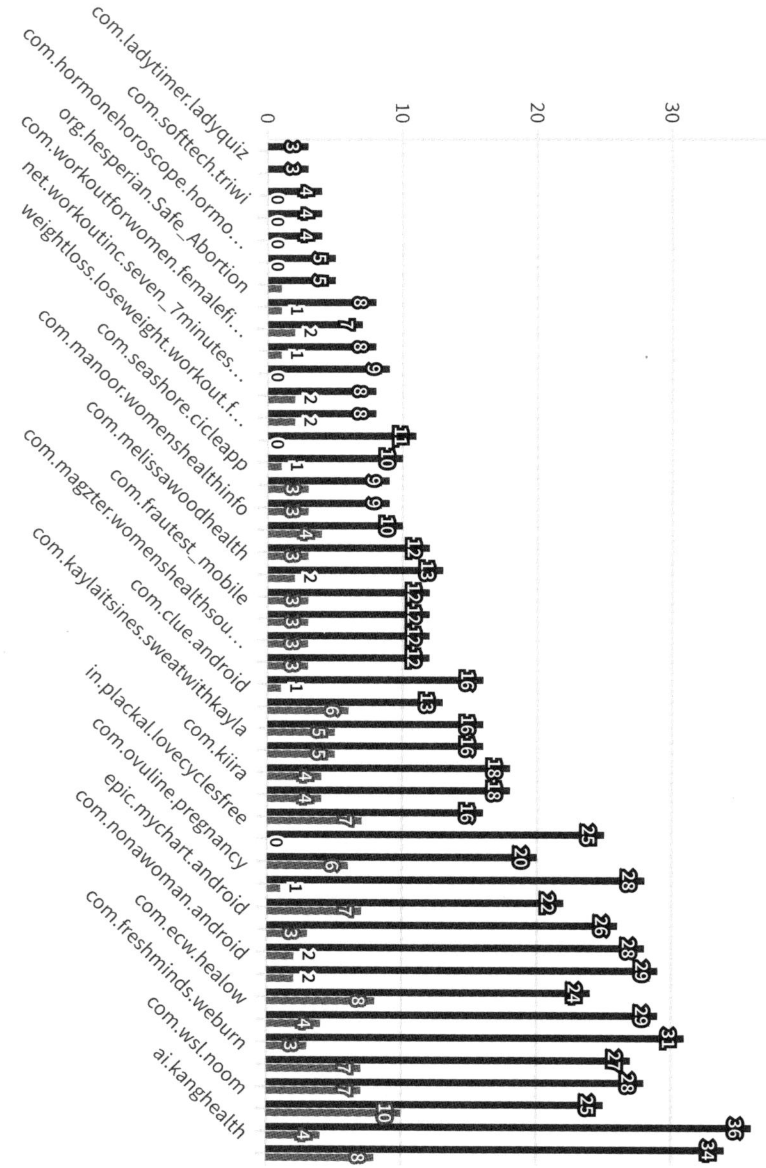

female health apps, unknowingly agreeing to several other parties to circumvent proper use of their data.

Each female health app necessitates permission from its user to collect information, with varying degrees of intrusiveness. Some permissions, such as sharing precise location data, unauthorised file downloads, audio recording, and reading call logs, can be deemed more invasive than others. For our research purposes, as depicted in Figure 4, permission counts are represented in black, and per-

Figure 4 Apps and their requested permissions.

missions categorized as particularly invasive are visually distinguished with a grey colour. Although the degree of intrusiveness is mostly subjective and may vary per user, it's worthwhile to wonder why some of these FemTech apps need access to our locations, contacts, or even our microphones. These permissions seem far from relevant to establishing female health—we can clearly state that this conflicts with how the apps typically market themselves to their consumers. In recent years, there has been a call to overcome the prevalent 'data anxiety', meaning a fear of sharing personal health information as a collective. While I wholeheartedly agree with this assertion and advocate data harvesting to unveil previously unnoticed insights, of which the medical field has many, it's become clear that the domain of female health confirms the legitimacy of data privacy concerns. Whether it's about pregnancy or user profiling and product recommendation, these apps do not show their users just how private their intimacy is and will be. The choice to work with third-party-trackers or to sell users' data to other platforms should naturally be condemned, preferably regulated. Unfortunately, as we've seen, these choices are part of a capitalist system we're all stuck in, a system that doesn't allow an app to be flaky, glitchy, or anything other than polished. An app like that would surely be deleted straight away. All books or resources on the creation of apps begin with: What business model will you have? What's the profit that'll keep the app running? This problematic and, alas, unavoidable mindset is indeed giving the development of ethical, non-oppressive apps a tough time. Although seeking true alternatives might seem almost impossible, it's imperative to keep researching the accountability of existing female health apps, considering the significance of their data.

Additionally, the question of free labour behind this data collection—for the app user is, of course, an unpaid source—brings with it a debate about the female body producing constant knowledge and subsequent products while still being endlessly used and freely consumed. In *Bleeding Data*, researchers Anastasia Siapka and Elisabetta Biasin underline how this new era of apps and data collection invites users to consider the work they freely provide:

'This unwaged labor can further be interpreted as gendered. Like the male breadwinners benefitting from their spouses' unpaid domestic labor, the industry capitalizing on FMT data and users' invisible labor is male-dominated, with some of the most popular FMTs having male Chief Executive Officers, while another one, Femm, was funded by "anti-abortion, anti-gay Catholic campaigners".'[7]

As the authors expand on a possibly more ethical redistribution of power and profit through the means of user compensation (that is, offering these bodies something in exchange for their data or knowledge), they strongly emphasise how *'evaluating the contractual nature of the pro-*

7 Anastasia Siapka and Elisabetta Biasin, "Bleeding Data: The Case of Fertility and Menstruation Tracking Apps," *Internet Policy Review* 10, no. 4 (2021).

vision of personal data as a service could be an interpretative way forward.'[8] However, this type of wealth redistribution fails to truly address the matter of safeguarding our privacy, our security and the prevention of transforming our bodies into mere commodities.

Caring for intimate data in the FemTech era is tricky in an overly connected, profit-driven industry. From perpetuating a reductive narrative around female health to selling abortion-related data to third parties, involving significant legal risk, these apps have done nothing to truly gain our trust. For example, Dr Maryam Mehrnezhad and Dr Teresa Almeida at Newcastle University show us in *Many Fertility Apps Not Exactly Fussy About Data Privacy* how notions around security, privacy, bias, and trust in IoT devices[9] are at the heart of their most recent research. This research, so they write, is *'calling for more adequate, lawful, and ethical processes when dealing with this data to ensure women get protection for the intimate information that is being collected by such technologies.'*[10] Additionally, Almeida and Mehrnezhad advise us to understand how marginalised user groups can shape what cybersecurity and privacy in these technologies can look like. But, we can wonder, even if privacy and security *were* respected, how useful would it be to analyse these platforms, if they only display the perspective of an ableist, female, white, fully functioning body? The notion that the creators of these female health applications harboured malicious intentions is not one that I endorse: it becomes increasingly harder to know whom to hold accountable for the perpetuation of stereotypical design or the dissemination of specific information. Considering the prevailing political climate and continuous expansion of the FemTech market, however, as well as its vast potential for societal influence, we have a social imperative to give back everything we observe to the user base of FemTech apps. Equally important is communicating such insights to prospective designers and developers who want to contribute to alternative, safe, and inclusive platforms in the future.

8 Siapka and Biasin, "Bleeding Data," 2021.

9 Abbreviation for Internet of Things. IoT devices are typically embedded with technology such as sensors and software, including mechanical and digital machines and consumer objects.

10 Newcastle University, "Many Fertility Apps Not Exactly Fussy about Data Privacy, Study Shows," Health Care In Europe, July 5, 2021.

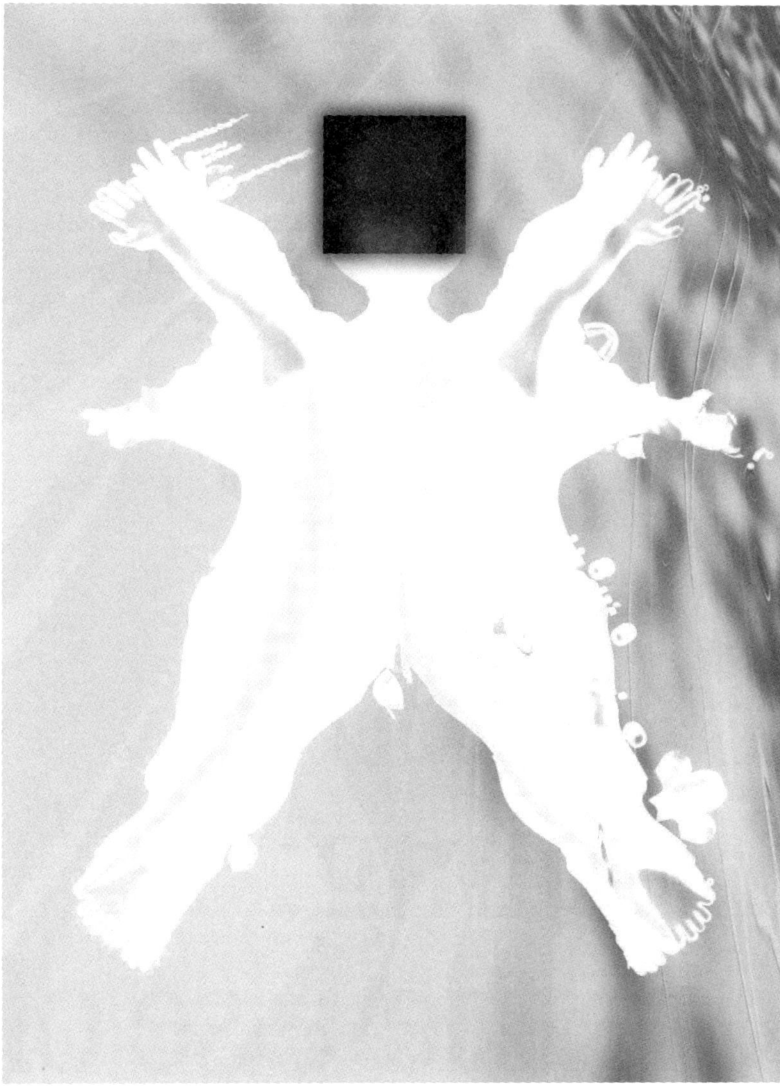

Figure 5 A valuable network opportunity by Morgane Billuart.

Chapter VI

Predictive Healing: On the Use of Algorithms in Fem Tech Apps

As I kept studying the ins and outs of data collection and app design, I would daydream about apps giving us what we truly *needed* rather than simply what we lacked. These fantasies painted a picture of a medical industry unlike our own, one that approached the study of our bodies and medicine completely different: offering highly-tailored pills and supplements catered to a person's specific requirements. An ideal system, it was, in my dreams, complemented by apps in which healing revolved around alleviating the stress and various forms of oppression our female bodies have to go through. Once I acknowledged the amount of work it would take to calculate and label each person's bodily experience, I realised that this dream might be both tedious and complex. Leaving that aside for a moment, let's fantasize some more, shall we? Into a future where technology can capture even the most intricate ideas and experiences. Into a world where FemTech apps finally grasp all the necessary details about our menstrual cycles, their forever fluctuating journey, and their outcome. A fantasy in which code is not just limited to the binary, and our daily input knows no bounds. Where algorithms and their predictions truly empower us to understand and care for our bodies.

As said before, many individuals wander online daily, endlessly seeking cures our current medical system has mostly failed to provide. While we've seen that it's still necessary to not completely turn your back on traditional medical institutions, anyone suffering from a chronic or misunderstood condition knows seeking help online is nothing short of survival. From my interview with the Instagram influencer behind PMDD Memes to my encounter with Rob in 't Zand and his startup *Health Thing* to writing this book, I can see a pattern of similar attempts. We all wish to create a community and build a support system by collecting our experiences and mutual concerns. In this, we merely want to be understood, aided, and share lessons with each other. Our collective view is pretty straightforward: the internet serves as a repository for all the knowledge we need to acquire. All one has to do is gather and present it. This is, perhaps, another comforting, almost naive illusion—one that means placing our faith in technology's ability to compute the unknown, where digital tools finally assist us in ways we previously couldn't support one another.

These past years, the use of algorithms in FemTech apps has made it possible to track menstrual cycles, fertility, and ovulation, as well as predict and diagnose various health conditions. Health apps, generally speaking —but also specifically FemTech—present themselves as a support structure in response to a need the medical institution failed to address. Although the healthcare system isn't just one monolith that can be easily criticised, it's fair to state that affordable, attentive, and *effective* care within female reproductive health is quite scarce. As a result, in a world where health practitioners are overworked, patients are misunderstood and unheard—certain promises of a more optimal, faster, and less biased health care seem very attractive. Recent discoveries within the humanities, however, have demonstrated that the use of these new health technologies doesn't just provide us with knowledge but also reinforces binary (gender) structures, turning what we wanted to be *cures* into cultural *artefacts*. Currently, the research focusing on the consequences of algorithms in our lives primarily investigates the day-to-day data we feed our machines. Algorithms behind platforms such as Netflix, Facebook, and YouTube are designed to keep us hooked, and they do. If we envision the future of digital healthcare as a large *hub*, a platform for discussion and exchange not unlike social media, then how can we guarantee the agenda behind this new format won't succumb to the same evil patterns currently constraining us?

Algorithms in FemTech Apps: In Between Values and Interests

Even though algorithms are ever-present in our lives—from the Spotify music in our ears to every product purchased online—their study seems overcomplicated, too cryptic for just anyone to comprehend. If they appear solely applicable (and thus understood) through the technologies they facilitate, they also shape culture, effectively moulding our society. As argued by Andreas Birkbak and Hjalmar Bang Carlsen in their book *Algorithmic Life*, *'the advantage of identifying and testing the ordering principles of [...] algorithms is that it becomes clear that they constitute specific interventions with various consequences.'*[1] In studying these algorithms, we can reveal their inner workings and examine each individual's role in shaping such an industry. How, for example, are our online habits formed? Indeed, due to the everyday utilisation of digital platforms, these tools pretend to 'magically' control our human needs and preferences. The algorithm knows what

1 Louise Amoore and Volha Piotukh (eds.), *Algorithmic Life: Calculative Devices in the Age of Big Data* (London: Routledge, 2016), 28.

you want. The algorithm knows what you need. Or does it? Critical research in algorithms often focuses on the data collection of 'innocent' details of our lives (again, our music taste or our favourite food) and wonders how these insights could still generate dangerous digital curations. For, yes, our love for vegan sushi or Post Malone might seem harmless, but when we shift this towards data regarding our physical or mental health, the risks are much, much higher.

In *Power Through the Algorithm*, David Beer emphasised how the movement toward Web 2.0 facilitated a sense of collaboration on the web, enabling users to get involved and generate content themselves.[2] Because of this, the medical institutions that once held a hegemonic power over knowledge production became criticised and rightfully questioned. As we've seen in previous chapters, this e-engagement in female health gave rise to a new generation of bloggers, YouTubers, forums, and holistic communities. Thanks to those individuals and their shared experiences, the internet started overturning the lack of understanding and support in the medical world. Using these gaps—perhaps as an excuse?—health apps and the broader digital health revolution zoom in on these issues, promising users a more specific rendering of their experiences while attempting to collect (and profit) from them. Such an enterprise, though, couldn't just be executed by the *human* brain. Due to the ever-expanding amount of work and patients to treat, the medical field started getting more and more invested in how technology could support diagnosing (and curing) our bodies. In *Ideal Algorithms in Healthcare*, researchers Tyler J. Loftus and Patrick J. Tighe underlined that *'the breadth and complexity of human disease confer unique challenges in clinical decision-making'*,[3] emphasising how, by contrast, *'high-complexity and high-volume data can be parsed by machine learning applications with relative ease.'*[4] Indeed, the use of such technology has been shown to potentially improve patient outcomes drastically. From handling administrative tasks to actively diagnosing disease, algorithms and machine learning can propose treatments faster and more effectively, especially as technology continues to improve. Machines can be wrong, you say? Of course. But then, humans and their institutions are also known to make mistakes frequently.[5] Seeing all of this, and mostly the desperate need for fast and well-rendered diagnosis, machine learning tools are an opportunity to produce more valuable, highly-needed knowledge and to optimise care within the industry.

At first glance, the speculative platform my peers and I dreamt of—the one that collects every individual's information to render something new—isn't so different from the digital health revolution and the goals set for algorithms in those apps. In her article *How AI Can Em-*

2 David Beer, "Power Through the Algorithm? Participatory Web Cultures and the Technological Unconscious," *New Media & Society - NEW MEDIA SOC* 11 (September 7, 2009): 985–1002.

3 Tyler J. Loftus et al., "Ideal Algorithms in Healthcare: Explainable, Dynamic, Precise, Autonomous, Fair, and Reproducible," *PLOS Digital Health*, January 18, 2022.

4 Loftus, "Ideal Algorithms," 2022.

5 Thi Ngoc Trang Tran et al., "Recommender Systems in the Healthcare Domain: State-of-the-Art and Research Issues," *Journal of Intelligent Information Systems* 57, no. 1 (August 1, 2021): 171–201.

power Women's Health, Dr Nicky Keay agrees with this. *'AI techniques'*, she says, *'can provide a way to combine personal clinical data with a medical understanding of female hormone networks.'* What's more: *'rather than "artificial" intelligence, it is more a case of "augmented" medical intelligence.'*[6] Numerous other papers indeed suggest that the use of these tools in the medical field generates a more accurate and precise diagnosis for those suffering from complex conditions. For example, in the study led in 2022, *Machine Learning Classifies Premenstrual Disorder*, researchers show how new technologies and data-driven methods can aid in analysing the brain and bodily experiences of those with Premenstrual Dysphoric Disorder or PMDD. In this study, the scientists merged meticulous neuroimaging datasets and a machine-learning technique to examine whether variances in brain morphology could be used to differentiate between women diagnosed with PMDD and the control group, which were mixed together.[7] In doing so, the research generated findings otherwise invisible or hard to locate, meaning the researchers could now move forward with more precision and accuracy, ultimately facilitating an official recognition of the condition; no small feat. While perhaps these advancements do not lead to an immediate practical change in the everyday life of PMDD sufferers, they are, nevertheless, propelling forward the recognition of a condition previously disregarded.

This recent research, showing us a glorious time in history when everything seemed quantifiable, also stipulates certain risks—especially once AI enters the picture. In *Artificial Intelligence in Female Reproductive Function*, Zhiyi Chen MD underlines that if *'AI was regarded as an efficient and reliable method to aid diagnosis, treatment, and prognosis in the medical field, it remains complex to seek for a "universal" or "global" agreement on how well should our bodies feel.'*[8] At the heart of every argument towards a big data-health revolution or the collection of menstruating bodies' experiences lies an enormous knowledge gap, waiting to be filled. For women's participation in clinical research was, and still is, scarce indeed. This past exclusion of our bodies and the instead standardised male figure is a reality that enabled the development of products, drugs, and assumptions about how female bodies should react, feel or behave. Only since the 1990s have certain laws and policies been (barely) adjusted, leaving our current medical system somehow *still* clueless about dealing with marginalised, other-than-male bodies. Seeing this massive blind spot sadly persisting, enlightenment through the use of machines and AI presented itself as a brand-new, promising ray of light. One that I, for one, gladly signed up for, and even encouraged many others to do so as well. After all, who doesn't wish to participate in the making of tomorrow's newest technologies, becoming a piece of a puzzle soon to be solved, becoming part of the solution?

6 Kirsty Rigg, "How AI Can Empower Women's Health," HT World, August 31, 2022.

7 SciLifeLab, "Machine Learning Classifies Premenstrual Dysphoric Disorder in Terms of Grey Matter Structure," SciLifeLab, November 9, 2022.

8 Zhiyi Chen et al., "Artificial Intelligence in the Assessment of Female Reproductive Function Using Ultrasound: A Review," *Journal of Ultrasound in Medicine* 41, no. 6 (June 1, 2022): 1343–53.

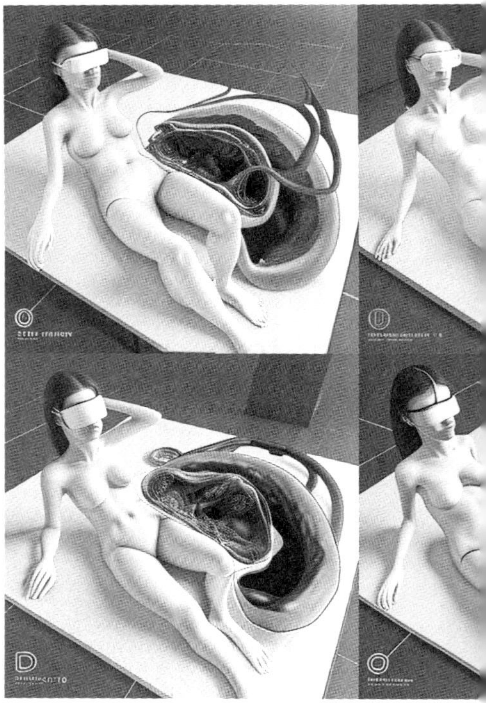

Figure 1 MidJourney prompt, '3D Model, Medical diagnosis rendering PMDD'.

Thanks to the popularisation of digital devices, online reviews, and other technological practices, sharing daily experiences and health-related data quickly became natural. However, this recent interest in life's computation isn't just guided by a desire to include and help marginalised groups; it's also an opportunity to capitalise on one of people's most fundamental needs: healthcare. As suggested by Statista, in 2021, artificial intelligence in the healthcare market was worth about 11 billion U.S. dollars, projected to be almost 188 billion U.S. dollars by 2030.[9] Specifically within the field of FemTech, AI Integration has pushed market growth annually by 15 per cent, promising a bright future indeed. Thankfully, researchers continue to study the many implications accompanying this fast expansion of computational and predictive tools. By doing so, an emphasis is put on the many financial (commercial) gains made from these developments: '*This sector will continue to attract a lot of new players and companies with varying standards of ethics, excellence, and quality.*'[10]

It's important, however, to differentiate between the development of such technology within hospitals, labs, and research institutes on the one hand, and those found in the digital health apps on the other. Although

9 Conor Stewart, "AI in Healthcare Market Size Worldwide 2021-2030," Statista Study, August 2022.

10 Karim Lekadir, University of Barcelona Department of Mathematics and Computer Science, Artificial et al., "Artificial Intelligence in Healthcare. Applications, Risks, and Ethical and Societal Impacts," May 2022.

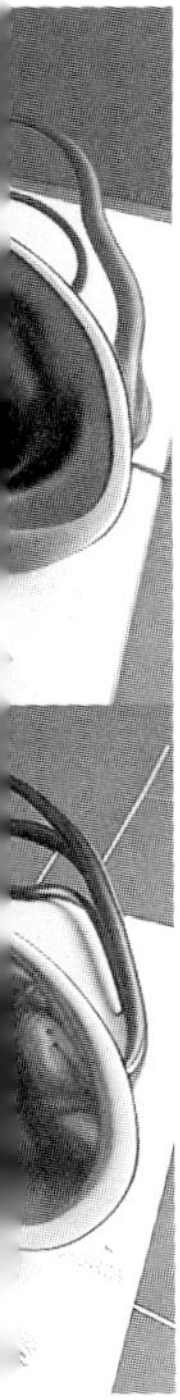

they seem interconnected, one should view a five-year research project on image recognition for breast cancer and a user-centred data analysis made from a few insights put into a mobile phone every other day. Coming back to *Power through the Algorithm* by Beer, who claims that *'computer scientists understand algorithms in terms of "rules"'*, but also that *'these rules are far different from the sorts of rules that human scientists have dealt with over the decades'.*[11] And, yes. Most research projects previously discussed on PMDD, PCOS, or endometriosis are funded and executed on a larger scale and timeframe. Therefore, they can lead to an in-depth analysis of what these conditions entail exactly, plus how to deal with them in a precise, highly clinical way. When we look at the tools FemTech apps work with, though, the algorithms and machine learning tools hidden in our devices, we see a very different kind of analysis. Their funding and remuneration systems also differ: the need for apps to produce and generate business models often implies that their design setup isn't solely informative, but rather more *suggestive*.

11 Beer, "Power Through the Algorithm?," 2009.

Many of these FemTech apps have, over the past years, declared an intention to not only display a brief overview of ovulation and fertility spikes, but also to collect as much information as possible about female health. In an email to VentureBeat, Flo founder and president Yuri Gurski wrote that *there are over fifty [female health] symptoms to track, and this number is likely to double in the future.*

Suddenly, these precise analyses made possible by mobile technology have become a golden goose, and the devices— way closer to the everyday life of female bodies than the medical field could ever be—are their golden eggs. After all, following the expansion of online forums and quantified self-habits, it's not a far stretch for smartphone users to start putting their daily flows and habits into the database of an app such as Flo. Slowly but surely, the app has made its way out in the world, and then suddenly, a gigantic pool of people, habits, and symptoms started to co-habit on the platform. In *Flo Health: Big Data in FemTech*, student Patric Cao sees the value creation behind these companies growing at an exponential rate: *'Flo Health has a proprietary data asset that follows 100M historical users for 7 years linking key discrete health data points to concrete health outcomes.'*[12]

12 Patric Cao, "Flo Health: Big Data in 'FemTech,'" Harvard Edu (blog), October 3, 2022.

With such an expansive collection of information, plus the proper tools, Flo has developed new features and predictions on their app, currently proposing paid membership with features such as *Health 360*, a complete package for more insights and analysis of one's cycles. Taking these developments and technological improvements aboard, Flo emphasised its commitment to the use of 'gold-standard diagnostic algorithms' to analyse data points and evaluate disease risks by measuring them against their large database. Does this sound a bit like our earlier dream of online communities having access to all the knowledge out there in the world? Why, yes! Technologies' powers seem to be used well here. And, with users, apps, and medical experts aligned, the possibilities for filling in knowledge gaps and craters in the fickle landscape of female health are endless.

Digital Health Speculations: Seeing Through the Black Box

Statistics: a collection of information shown in numbers.[13]

Algorithms: a set of rules that must be followed when solving a particular problem.[14]

Machine Learning: a type of artificial intelligence in which computers use huge amounts of data to learn how to do tasks rather than being programmed to do them.[15]

Let's look at the difference between self-analysis, collective knowledge, medical analysis, and data-rendered diagnosis when talking about FemTech apps. As said in the earlier chapter *Gathering the Wounded's Traces*, self-tracking and peer-to-peer recommendation are some of the most ancient ways to heal oneself and to share knowledge. Although these might not strictly be 'science', these techniques were a way for individuals to care for each other throughout history. Nowadays, products recommended by other members in online communities are not based on a careful analysis of individuals' similarities and differences, but rather on the

13 "Statistics," in: *Oxford Dictionary*. Oxford, n.d.

14 "Algorithm," in: *Oxford Dictionary*. Oxford, n.d.

15 "Machine Learning," in: *Oxford Dictionary*. Oxford, n.d.

fragile and ever-changing belief that what has worked for one person might also work for another. These exchanges between communities—even more so online—are, to a certain extent, collective embodied knowledge. A precious and valid kind of knowledge, for sure, yet also a somewhat volatile one, with potential side effects. I still think about the time I recommended using Boric Acid against yeast infections. Inserting such a capsule into a vagina can be toxic, so I always insisted that *'I just read this somewhere. Please be careful. Also, I'm not a doctor.'* Here's hoping what has helped me will help all of us. To be honest, I'd much rather put my faith in a diagnosis than run through millions of datasets to find the exact solution me and my peers need. The thought of such a predictive tool appears to me less naive, more specific; therefore becoming a potential guide on the muddy road towards healing.

Research statistics in the medical field are, of course, also a helpful guide towards better understanding our bodies' reactions to a certain type of drug. Collecting this information was first labelled as simply 'knowledge', then later became what made possible the commercialisation of products sold to consumers. While there's no guarantee that a drug will work for someone, the statistical analysis of a product from a similar pool of patients increases a positive outcome. Before algorithms and machine learning were even known to healthcare, statistical methods were used to oversee patient treatments. These statistics have been studied and used for over a thousand years, with the first writings dating back to... yep, the 8th century. At its core, the principles of statistics come down to the following questions: What can we learn about a topic from a set pool of individuals? What are the patterns and differences observed? The later use of algorithms and machine learning in health-related apps was designed to make repeatable predictions by finding patterns within data. In itself, algorithmic uses and machine learning concerning female health aren't far removed from what already exists: a more or less assumed and normative knowledge about our bodies. The only difference, really, is the computational power of such tools. If before (general) observations could only be made for a specific group of individuals, an ideal machine learning program would run studies on a *planetary* scale and shed light on all things never seen before. We could, then, speak of a shift from general knowledge to one of precise predictions, almost mechanical in nature.

Now, *how* exactly can these computers and their analytical power help us uncover all of these detailed observations? A question the great bosses behind the digital health agenda are undoubtedly asking themselves. The answer to this depends on whom you ask: the patient, the app provider, or the medical institution. For example, when browsing Reddit conversations on PMDD, Endometriosis, and other conditions, one observes a frustration with not being understood, listened to, or, in general, not fitting the mould our society tries to place us in. Users seek understanding and patience while hoping for pain and discomfort to, finally, be understood. An issue that no highly accurate prediction for pills or drugs could easily solve: one cannot package a sympathetic ear into a box and sell it. When FemTech enterprise collects data about our mental and physical experiences, they hope to smooth over any questions about how our bodies function. This datafication should be regarded with criticism, however, as these processes have proven to simultaneously measure, manipulate, and *monetise* online human behaviour—which we've seen at length in previous chapters. A more philosophical paradox seems to appear instead: how can we render something through machines that has not been previously acknowledged or even perceived? If medical misogyny and female pain have always been ignored, how can these digital tools help us break the chains?

Looking beyond just the world of digital health, we see a systemic belief regarding technology and its ability to reveal what cannot be seen, and what is yet to be discovered. *The computer eye sees what the human can not.* In physics, computational simulations allow us to visualise black holes. In sci-fi, the mini-series Devs introduced a visual, almost tangible experience of Jesus Christ rendered through specific mathematical formulas. In healthcare, researchers are still trying to fix historical shortcomings, enhancing our understanding of the human (female) body. But this magical black box of a machine they want to employ might prove rather problematic. In *What Algorithms Want*, Ed Finn argues for an in-depth study of what *isn't* visible in machines, underlying how *'the implementation gap is the most important thing we need to know, and the thing we most frequently misunderstand, about algorithmic systems.'*[16] Furthermore, he stresses, the mystical notion of computation as a kind of *'universal truth'* should be reviewed, for often we *'see this faith in computation invoked repeatedly at the intersection of algorithms and culture.'*[17] Finn underlines how careful we should be in giving *too* much credit to these machines, as we not only create these supportive environments, but they, in turn, create us.[18]

Participating in these healthcare computations means transforming our daily experiences into a series of formulas. The various pinpoints of these computations aren't wholly transparent, and the black box, that prime idea of a machine smarter than us, is regarded as so complex that its workings aren't interpretable to humans, often

16 Ed Finn, *What Algorithms Want: Imagination in the Age of Computing* (Cambridge: MIT Press, 2018), 2.

17 Finn, *What Algorithms Want*, 2018, 9.

18 Finn, *What Algorithms Want*, 2018, 50, 37.

leaving us clueless about the principles behind its freshly gathered knowledge. *Thank you, dear, but how exactly did you come about this?* While the mechanisms of this machine seem slowly more palpable over time, the actual logic behind a black box and its predictions remains unresolved. Interestingly enough, many FemTech app leaders argue that in their revolution, it's the female body that's the true mystery. As Oriana Kraft argues in her article *FemTech Startups*, *'hormones are core to women's reproductive and general health, yet they remain a black box.'*[19] What this demonstrates is that at the heart of this revolution, a desire for change exists, an ideology that wants to compute the body, rendering its rules and patterns visible through data, thus showing these bodily experiences are real, something that can be healed. The female body is a computable object, this revolution shouts at us. And yet, by attempting to make these bodies more 'transparent', FemTech apps use mechanisms of computation that are, as seen, not always comprehensive, logical, or even fair. Furthermore—repeating ourselves, but it needs to be said—they draw their conclusions with a very *specific* (aka: standard) female body in mind.

19 Oriana Kraft, "FemTech Startups Innovating Hormonal Health," FemTechnology.org, March 24, 2022.

Feeding Diversity: The Prerequisite of Fair Predictive Technologies

Whether we're talking about the medical field or other, criticism of data collection often revolves around the *bias* rooted within these systems, not to mention the less-than-diverse pool of data participants. But, as Louise Amoore and Volha Piotukh argue in Algorithmic Life, a world filled with openness and interconnectedness leads to the realisation of a common good: all of us working towards freeing each other. Empowering individuals to share their knowledge plays a crucial role in creating this worldview where everyone benefits.[20] Unfortunately, many of these tools are, of course, not accessible to some people, with

20 Amoore, *Algorithmic Life*, 2016.

participants in data studies effectively rendering it into an elitist, normative research. As suggested in *The Downside of Machine Learning in Health Care*, Marzyeh Ghassemi suggests a cautious attitude towards AI in medicine. *'If used carefully,'* she tells us, *'this technology could improve performance in health care and potentially reduce inequities, but if we're not careful, technology could worsen care.'*[21] She emphasises the need to get our hands on *'better data'*, reminding us how biases could worsen the (already frail) promises of the digital health revolution. Ghassemi not only points out the issues regarding possible faulty information being generated, but also argues that the healthcare industry, to get better data, should incentivise its broader collection—in essence, to get even more of it—preferably in the most inclusive way. These directives should also be considered when applied specifically to the FemTech industry, even though debates around surveillance and data privacy might hinder this.

Research on the problematic biases within artificial intelligence, something most of us already know about, has a slightly different focus when looking at health care. While most of the studies around this underline AI's potential to improve patient outcomes drastically, they also warn us about the potential disasters of data not being rendered properly. Katherine J. Igoe sees in *Algorithmic Bias in Health Care* how *'algorithmic bias can have devastating effects on people of color at all points in the health care process, from triaging their illnesses to the quality of care they receive.'*[22] Furthermore, Igoe says, these AI systems have already failed minorities, specifically Black communities, by completely disregarding their absence in risk-prediction data sets—also think of self-driving cars not recognising a Black person, thus being at risk of running them over. In AI healthcare, as a result of a lack of Black patients within the studies, the algorithm disqualified them from receiving extra care, thinking that their absence meant a reduced necessity for care, instead of what it really was: a limited access to resources, to actually *finding* this care.[23] What's more, the bias already set in these health care algorithms often never gets fixed, instead implementing itself into newer models over and over, thus perpetuating faulty judgment by humans and its own bias. Indeed, by making predictions and possible suggestions based on teachings from the past—information that was never proven to be *right*—it becomes near impossible not to replicate false patterns, especially if the same parties organise the design and implementation of these technologies. In *Artificial Intelligence in Healthcare*, Karim Lekadir from the University of Barcelona suggests something similar, emphasising that, *'if not properly implemented, evaluated and regulated, future AI solutions could embed and even amplify the systemic disparities and human biases that contribute to healthcare inequities.'*[24] And in the FemTech industry? All of their predictions and recommendations seem rather dangerous if they

21 Steve Nadis, "The Downside of Machine Learning in Health Care," News MIT, February 1, 2022.

22 Katherine J. Igoe, "Algorithmic Bias in Health Care Exacerbates Social Inequities – How to Prevent It," Harvard School of Public Health (blog), March 12, 2021.

23 Igoe, "Algorithmic Bias in Health Care," 2021.

24 Lekadir, "Artificial Intelligence in Healthcare," 2022.

online refer to the normative body: a white, privileged, and cisgender female. While these apps are developing many features to try and create a complex layering of our bodily experiences, they should also include data from an inclusive group of individuals before they can even claim their knowledge as 'real'.

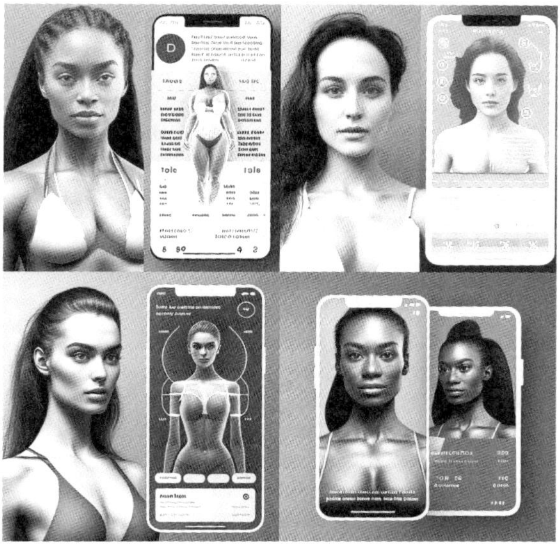

Figure 2 MidJourney prompt: 'Hyper-realistic FemTech apps, inclusive and diverse'.

Bethany Corbin sees in *Digital Micro-Aggressions and Discrimination* that FemTech apps often convey a very singular idea of what it means to have control over one's body, instead suggesting they produce severely flawed views on body conformity. Corbin furthermore argues that *'digital products are consistently telling women what their biology should be, what their reproductive goals should be, and what their sexual activity and preferences should be.'*[25] Consequently, she raises concerns about how the technology industry can address and rectify these flawed assumptions, their design shortcomings, and all the corporate policies negatively impacting FemTech. What can be done to prevent the perpetuation of stereotypes and marginalisation within the female-bodied population? With this, we see Corbin worrying about the nature of possible solutions, warning that these will require a fundamental shift in how society perceives its consumers. At the core of Corbin's research, she asks us to wonder how, as we feed machines with data, we unknowingly participate in the general othering of women. Corbin also rightfully underlines that while these technologies have the potential to generate more visibility and knowledge around intersex and non-binary bodies, they, as of yet, seem to

25 Bethany Corbin, "Digital Micro-Aggressions and Discrimination: FemTech and the 'Othering' of Women," Nova Law Review, Vol. 44, 2020.

ignore their presence instead, along with the depth of their experiences.

Let us, then, entertain ourselves with some speculation. What could be a fair use of algorithms in the healthcare industry, specifically within FemTech? The *Fair Machine Learning in Healthcare* research by Qizhang Feng and others explores how the bias happening at each point in the research can be identified and corrected. These researchers underline, for example, how the initial data collection might imply structural biases, particularly *'when the sample size of a demographic group is smaller than that of other groups'.*[26] To resolve these issues, the researchers suggest, attention should be paid to collecting information on exactly these missing demographics, rendering them visible once more. Additionally, one could propose a different way of looking at data collection: something that can support health practitioners and users, but that isn't necessarily a fundamental truth. As José van Dijck sees it, *'datafication enthusiasts also often assume a self-evident relationship between data and people, subsequently interpreting aggregated data to predict individual behavior.'*[27] While these correlations one assumes while reading data might mean no harm, they can distinctly hurt our previously sketched stereotypes and blind spots. Simultaneously, as Corbin saw it, users expecting health apps to offer them reliable, thoroughly researched knowledge shouldn't forget that the processes of datafication and 'life mining' are deeply rooted in (often false) ideological presumptions that, in turn, confirm social norms.[28]

Returning to the research *Ideal Algorithms in Healthcare*, we can see Tyler J. Loftus and his team making an extensive list of all the things researchers and companies should consider when generating new healthcare knowledge. In their conclusion, they propose an ideal algorithm with six requirements represented in the following checklist: *'explainable, dynamic, precise, autonomous, fair, and reproducible'.* By achieving these objectives, they continue, *healthcare algorithms confer maximum potential benefits to patients, clinicians, and investigators.'*[29] While this seems like a rather complex list of prerequisites, what we have learned in this chapter shows how they should be seen as referential methods, necessary to avoid falling into dangerous traps in thinking about our bodies. Applying this to the field of FemTech, Corbin asks us to consider a few ways to 'fix' FemTech's analysis whenever it's reductive. *'FemTech products'*, she says, *'should be heavily vetted by diverse consumer groups before launch. While several FemTech companies currently do this, some companies nonetheless feel pressure to rush to market, and do not ensure adequate testing among representative consumers.'*[30]

Again, let us look at what these apps and algorithms can do for us in terms of filling in knowledge gaps, rather than pretending they hold an absolute truth. Perhaps we can conduct an in-depth study of all the different kinds

26 Qizhang Feng, Mengnan Du, Na Zou and Xia Hu, "Fair Machine Learning in Healthcare: A Review," arXiv, 2022.

27 José Van Dijck, "Datafication, Dataism and Dataveillance: Big Data Between Scientific Paradigm and Ideology," Surveillance & Society 12 (May 9, 2014).

28 Van Dijck, "Datafication," 2014.

29 Loftus, "Ideal Algorithms," 2022.

30 Corbin, "Digital Micro-Aggressions," 2020.

of participants using the FemTech apps? In pinpointing exactly who the majorities and the minorities are, these apps could paint a more realistic landscape of female bodies', making transparent the various information clusters out there, plus their disparities. Thus, instead of perpetuating harmful general notes around bodies, they could be the ones that show each body as culturally different. We are not being unnecessarily hard on FemTech apps: it is precisely *because* they hold such great potential that they should be critically studied. The future of fair, comprehensive female health also cannot exist without smoothing over every knowledge gap we can find–something we've made clear here. Still, bridging these gaps is far from the only thing needed. As previously seen, a more systemic, societal change needs to happen. If fair and inclusive data collection is the goal, many more challenges come to mind when considering ethical healthcare predictions. Coming back to Ed Finn's book *What Algorithms Want*, he shows us how important it is to acknowledge that this knowledge gap isn't quite the same as the glitches, crashes, or any other indicators of dysfunctional computational systems.[31] By underlying the differences between those terms, Finn invites us to wonder how we can still consider those things that, in essence, are hard to grasp, and perhaps will never be computable. Fundamentally, this questions whether we can rely on machines to better understand the complexity of human experiences and our own bodies, or not.

In their book *Pattern Discrimination*, Clemens Apprich, Florian Cramer, Wendy Hui Kyong Chun, and Hito Steyerl look at different patterns and biases created in our ever-more-expanding digital, computational world. They suggest a speculative future where data-driven politics are taken seriously and *'systems that acknowledge the fundamental fluidity of identity'* exist.[32] Also criticising the power dynamics behind these operations, they scrutinise who gets to choose these data-driven methods, and what sort of real consequences their interpretations have. Similar ideologies are found in feminist literature, those who wish to embrace the natural essence of fluidity, acknowledging the unquantifiable now often still defined as a 'glitch', wondering what potential this glitchy fluidity has as a political statement. (For it is political not to be fully optimal, as we have seen, and thus the circle is round. Or should we say: cycle?) The glitch shows that, just like our bodies, machines also never run perfectly. Perhaps the trouble these algorithms, black boxes, machines and apps currently have in capturing our bodies' perfect imperfections should be viewed as growing pains, ones we should manage and dissect closely. Critically managing these new platforms as well as possible enables us to include more unheard voices, to feed the debate more diverse perspectives on what the future of female health can and *should* look like. While further use of intelligent

31 Finn, What Algorithms Want, 2018, 50.

32 Clemens Apprich et al., Pattern Discrimination (Minnesota: University of Minnesota Press, 2018), 12.

systems might appear inevitable, a constant re-evaluation of their inner workings and hidden agendas remains not only vital, but also the leading strategy in demanding more equitable designs in the future.

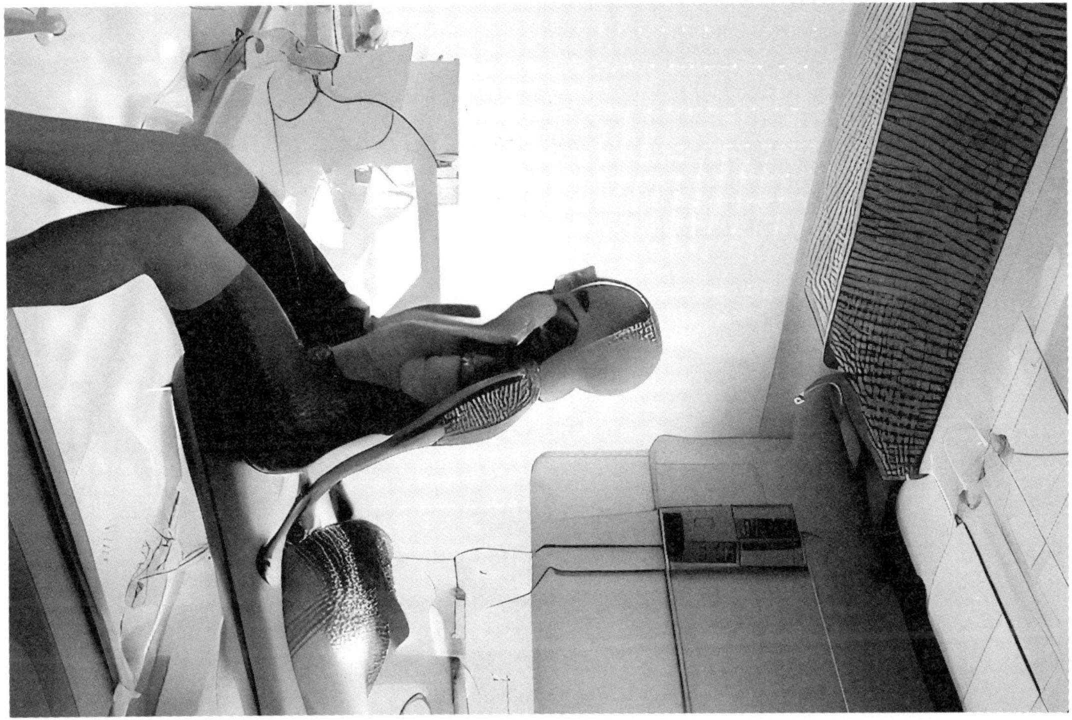

Figure 3 Cyberpunk Generator, 'Femtech app health inclusive UI'.

Chapter VII

The Glitch Ideology and the Potentiality of Contingency with Carmen Hines

In the final stages of this book, I wasn't sure if its conclusion needed a recap of all the themes discussed, or rather a wrap-up promising brighter days for the future of female health. What I did know, however, is that this book could have never happened without the other books I researched, the conversations I've had, and the emotional support of the amazing women who surrounded me constantly. Whether these were friends, collaborators, strangers, remote researchers, or online intellectuals, their experiences and anecdotes gave me the strength and the courage to keep writing when I felt incapable of studying such an immense, complex, and triggering topic. Although I cannot mention all of their names here, this last chapter is an attempt to render a conversation I myself wished I had heard or been invited to sooner.

While writing this book, in my quest for more collaborators, I had the pleasure to come across Carmen Lael Hines, a young curator and thinker who, at the time, lived in Vienna as well. Barely could I contain my joy when Carmen and I started to exchange, produce, and brainstorm about our research, whether it was about FemTech, automation, seduction, pods, or love (yes, love). To befriend a woman my age with similar ambitions and topics of fascination is something I hadn't experienced before. This chapter is an opportunity to conduct a different kind of research on FemTech, instead engaging in an organic conversation about future designs, pathways to change, and much more.

The following paragraphs are snippets from Carmen Lael Hines' chapter: 'Natural Cycles: The Aesthetics and Architectures of FemTech' published in *Reality Harvester: Data After Nature* (Skoden, 2022).

Natural Cycles is one fertility and menstruation app in a growing industry broadly referred to as FemTech. Natural Cycles, founded in 2013, is spearheading what the start-up refers to as a technology of 'digital contraception,' becoming, in their words, 'one of the hottest and fastest growing startups in Sweden.' Somewhere between a tech start-up, pharmaceutical company, health service, and wellness facilitator – Natural Cycles offers a hormone-free form of contraception, and prides itself in being 'non-invasive', 'natural', 'alternative', and 'safe'. With a monthly fee of 9.99 euros a month + the purchase of a thermometer, it works through the use of an algorithm that calculates the window in a month a user is likely to be fertile, based on basal body temperature readings, menstrual cycle information and other biological data provided by the user including: the consistency of cervical mucus, or blood quantity (light, spotting or heavy). Based on this data, the app indicates when the user is ovulating and should either abstain from sex or use protection to prevent pregnancy. In 2018, it became the first app to be cleared for marketing as a contraceptive by the U.S. Food and Drug Administration (FDA) after being certified as a contraceptive in the European Union in 2017.

Though the app has been accredited by the FDA as a valid form of contraception, the accuracy and the efficacy of FMTs are heavily contested. Their unpredictability comes from the fact that to track basal body temperature correctly, the user must do so at the exact time every day, at the exact moment they wake up. Stress levels, or having a life that in the words of Diana Zuckermann (president of the National Centre for Health Research), is 'a bit complicated,' will certainly affect the efficiency of this form of contraception. The app received profoundly bad press in 2017 when a study reported that in the largest hospital in Stockholm, 37 out of 668 women who underwent abortions there had been using Natural Cycles as a contraceptive when they became pregnant. The CDC generally advises that 'fertility awareness methods' which Natural Cycles attests to optimizing through machine learning, can have a failure rate of up to 23%.

The FDA suggests that the app shouldn't be used by individuals for whom pregnancy would be a 'major risk' to the mother. The app would be ideal for users who intend on getting pregnant in the next few years, or for whom getting pregnant would not necessarily be catastrophic. As has been investigated by research groups and journalists, Natural Cycles was cleared through an FDA pathway for new types of low- to moderate-risk devices, a policy which has been argued to align far more with the desires of Big Pharma than for the benefit of public health. In other words, it received market authorization because it will not cause 'immediate risk'. What 'risk' entails, however, becomes troubling, subjective, and contingent on things such as class, age, and overall lifestyle. You will certainly not drop dead from inserting your daily temperature into an app. But as an effective form of contraception, OBGYNs and other reproductive health professionals, have expressed that its effectiveness is questionable, and hugely dependent on a user's lifestyle, and the regularity to which the user engages with the app itself.

It was this that motivated the 2018 lawsuit from the ASA, or Advertising Standards Authority, which claimed that attesting to the fact that the app was 'highly accurate' and a 'clinically tested alternative to birth control methods,' was inaccurate. The allegations were upheld and Natural Cycles was requested to remove said adverts. Perusing the website today, the same ideas are presented, but just in slightly different words, phrases like 'we are birth control, we are effective,' and through a particular kind of socialization suggested through the ad campaigns. What is not said, but rather suggested through aesthetics and visual culture.

Although fertility awareness methods are one of the least effective forms of contraception due to their extreme contingency, everything about the Natural Cycles media campaigns suggests the contrary. It is presented as profoundly safe, medically viable, comforting, and 'non-invasively' natural. Perusing the website, the language is that of a frantic defensiveness of its medical legitimacy, under the veil of a plethora of 'Cyclers,' or Natural Cycles influencers, sharing their experiences using the app, including familiar faces like *Love Island* finalist Montana Brown. Phrases like 'It made me feel more connected to myself and my body,' 'I was looking for something natural, hormone-free' and 'it taught me that alternatives are possible' circulate the hyper-saturated and styled webpage. The aesthetics are an explosion of 'wellness' typologies: house plants, candles, white sheets, silk pajamas, and so, so, many journals.

It becomes clear in researching the app, that the self-monitoring and regulatory lifestyle revealed in the adverts is not only a seductive media strategy, but necessary for the app to work. The contraception works is a user engages in detailed, routine self-calculation and consistent, daily input of data. The engagement with 'community affirmation' via paid influencers, which suggests transparency, authenticity, and honesty – is a strategy necessary to legitimize themselves as a contraception as effective as the pill, coil, or IUD. The necessity for users to engage in detailed self-monitorization and regulation, and the dangers if they do so otherwise, are not situated with resolution. This messiness is brushed under the rug, implied or nudged through the visual culture of their media campaigns that propose an aesthetics and architecture of calculability (in white and beige). This nudging evades and packages what is indeed an entangled, vulnerable architecture in constant dialogue with glitch *potential* – instead, the company suggests, and necessitates aspirational, glitchless world of #goddess life, a projection field of the social behaviors aligned with the logic that the company relies on to both make money and to function.

Poetics of Inconsistencies

(MORGANE) Let's dive into your work by underlying this concept of body contingency, often referred to as 'the glitch'. I, too, have explored this idea: how can we use an app to highlight the various pressures experienced by women? How can we showcase the dysfunction, not of an individual body, but of the system itself? While I find this notion captivating, acknowledging non-performativity is inherently dramatic. It's more of a compelling narrative to engage in individual managerialism—pushing ourselves into maximum efficiency—rather than recognising one's failures. Who would be willing to do that, focus on their own failing? It requires acknowledging one's inability to conform in the first place, which entails significant mental effort that many people cannot afford to invest, or simply choose not to. When contemplating the glitches in these apps, I wonder: what could drive such a design? What can it bring to one's life?

(CARMEN) That's a crucial question to consider, indeed. In the case of Natural Cycles, what you describe as 'failure' is really not that. It's just whatever exists outside of (data) calculability. Maybe you forget to put information into the app, maybe you're stressed, maybe you lose your thermometer on the train, maybe you had a one-night stand and forgot your thermometer at home. My investigation pushed me to consider how making contraception profit-oriented (the app Natural Cycles wants to help you prevent pregnancy, yet also wants to sell you stuff, red.) means that the potential for 'error' or 'glitch' is not presented with enough clarity. When you're claiming to provide something that can help people not get pregnant, this has the potential to mess with people's lives. But the problem may not be the fact that this technology exists, but that its interface design, as well as the profit orientations informing this design, approach the potential for error, glitch, or 'failure' in a rather problematic way: smoothing it over at every turn.

However, setting aside this specific case study, it might be too easy to assume every interface of for-profit apps (or even companies as a whole) promotes a perfectly performed subject. I think, in reality, that it's much more complex than this—some ad campaigns consciously market non-perfection and subjectivity. It aligns with what you mentioned about cognitive dissonance, the marketing strategy which says DON'T BUY THIS, so you buy it; think of the subversive marketing plant-based milk Oatly did quite successfully. There are instances where the idea of embracing glitches or failures can be used to sell the subject. It's an ongoing social criticism that goes beyond mere aspiration: right now, it revolves more around acknowledging the potential for failure, errors, mistakes, or even flirting with rebelliousness. I saw an advert recently that read something like: Hey babez, don't leave me on read. I wonder when 'glitchiness,' to use Legacy Russell's term, becomes another avenue for 'selling'.

Don't get me wrong... I love the glitch. In much of what I currently read, there is a sentiment about deliberately avoiding excessive perfection. It's a beautiful concept, but I struggle to find its actual presence or implementation in anything. It remains a beautiful ideology, yet it seems to lack tangible realisation. *(MORGANE)*

(CARMEN) Yes, I agree. I prefer 'contingency' to 'glitch'. Recently, I came across a proposal for sleep as a political alternative, but I find it difficult to embrace this idea fully. Starting a revolution simply through sleeping doesn't seem inspiring to me. Even Marx and Gramsci suggest the importance of productivity and intentional action for creating change. Changing things for the better is not about non-activity, but rather about forming a personal or collective practice—one not solely focused on finding solutions or pursuing individual goals. This is why I love working with you, Morgane, for instance, and writing or developing ideas together, supporting one another with navigating a precarious career in academia in our twenties. The productivity of this particular approach lies in the collective communication and decisions made by the subject(s), creating a different structure altogether.

Your perspective reminds me of a text recently discussing the different strategies employed by the left and the right. It raises the question of why people are drawn to choose the 'blue pill', and why they would want to stay in a system of suppression. I'm not suggesting that the political right has a superior story, but rather that they present a convenient one that offers comfort, a sense of reassurance. Something like, 'If you follow this path, everything will be fine.' When relating these concepts to the glitch, I wonder: why would people be interested in embracing such a doomed, imperfect statement? What does it mean to realise one's inability to conform to societal expectations, particularly when many individuals falsely believe they can meet those standards? At the end of the day, we all live in an ableist society. *(MORGANE)*

(CARMEN) Certainly! I can relate to that on a personal level. Quite often, I still struggle with the feeling of failure, whether in terms of my body, job, or relationships. It creates a sense of exclusion because I feel like everyone else seems to be participating in something, succeeding—which I am not. I guess this is one of the repercussions of the #GirlBoss hegemony.

I highly agree with the need for connection and a space to foster change and critical thinking. Having more options and platforms is crucial for people to share their fears, wonders, and questions. However, I find myself contemplating the challenges of creating such a platform, one that goes beyond a mere gathering space for knowledge and exchange. How extensive is the issue of 'finding solutions'? Is it solely a technical problem, or does it also have philosophical implications? *(MORGANE)*

(CARMEN) To go beyond the pursuit of optimisation, it's essential to look at the underlying politics and philosophical frameworks that drive individuals to prioritise optimisation. These technological tools, such as apps, phones, and other devices, result from various political, philosophical, and structural relationships that shape their development. They are not detached from these influences, but instead intertwined with them.

In my research, I came across Stefano Harney and Frederic Morton's recent book All Incomplete, which explores this concept. In the introduction by Denise Ferreira Da Silva, she presents a fascinating perspective on desire as the presence of a demand for choice. She also highlights the algorithm as the formal decision-making tool of logistical capitalism. However, this algorithm fails when confronted with a situation that exceeds its capacity, causing the process to halt when the input doesn't align with the available data. This notion raises exciting questions about the limitations of optimisation-driven systems and their potential for disruption when encountering scenarios beyond their scope. It invites us to reflect on the intricate relationship between desire, decision-making algorithms, and the constraints of logistical capitalism.

(MORGANE) It suggests that there are restrictions within the algorithms, correct?

(CARMEN) Basically, what they're saying is that the information, or input, is inserted into the algorithm's structure. The algorithm is designed with a predetermined architecture that determines where the input will be placed. As a result, the input is treated as an object, such as a woman, and the information is transformed into something else. In the context of (FemTech) apps, the input refers to the collective production of data.

(MORGANE) Yes, but let's consider an example of an app that aims to depict racial diversity or the lack thereof. For instance, let's say Clue and Flo point out that the app predominantly features white individuals, making up 99 per cent of the representation, while neglecting other racial groups. In essence, representing what is missing is not technically challenging but does need a shift in ideology.

(CARMEN) It seems like you're asking how we can develop a concrete strategy that addresses an abstract concept on a large scale. This requires questioning the formation of the neoliberal subject, which revolves around the idea of optimisation. It's challenging even to imagine this, because our relationship with technology often revolves around that very notion. However, this is where the text All Incomplete is helpful. There's a quote that resonates with this issue, asking, 'How can improvement occur without knowing the "what" and the "how"?' Essentially,

it delves into the philosophical purpose of these apps and how their intentions are carried out. It's not enough to simply attribute glitches to the apps and embrace them. There needs to be an intention to actively engage with a structure, whatever that might look like. Currently, the existing structure is built upon optimisation, the commodification of the body, and the enforced production of femininity. Truly changing this would require establishing a new definition of improvement, one that doesn't focus on predefined notions of self-betterment. Instead, we should create a cybernetic model of self-improvement based on collective aspirations.

(MORGANE)

What you're saying reminds me of a quote from Paul B. Preciado's book, Testo Junkie. Preciado asks whether we want to change the world and experience it with the same systems and sincerity we already possess, or if we prefer to alter our perception through the lens of beauty and the somatic filter. It raises the question of whether we want to see the world as it is and take action, or if we want to modify it. Technology and neoliberalism often focus on alteration, fixing oneself, changing perceptions, etc. In his book, Preciado shares his experience of taking testosterone, which made him feel more vibrant, sexually driven, and hungry. In a way, this represents an optimal state. As I was reading this book, I wondered: why wouldn't I pursue this, too? That's also something Preciado wonders, by asking the following question: 'Why isn't everyone using testosterone as a means of birth control to enhance vitality and desire?' At the same time, this vision is deeply dystopian, as it involves selecting the most 'optimal' versions of ourselves while disregarding everything else. What are our options?

(CARMEN)

While working on my chapter for 'Reality Harvester', I contemplated what a truly radical FemTech model could look like. I envisioned a scenario inspired by a quote from the CEO of Natural Cycles about implanted chips that constantly monitor body temperature —very cyborg, very sci-fi. Today, however, we can see ethical challenges arising from the intentions behind these FemTech apps, their capitalistic motives, and how they turn individuals into commodities. But what if the intention shifted? What if the aim was to create an informational and hackable system, rather than treating individuals as products? Complex questions, because they revolve around intentional choices regarding the desired framework to align with. Coming back to Paul B. Preciado: he's actively optimising himself, yes, but still within a structure that challenges the conventional notion of optimisation.

(MORGANE)

Let's imagine a health app to be released tomorrow, one claiming to reveal not how to become better or optimal, but how to support users in seeing possible glitches and inconsistencies. Then, the same question comes up: why would people choose to use such an app?

(CARMEN) I believe that people want to form solidarity. They want recognition.

(MORGANE) That's precisely why I believe that collective exchange and movement are necessary. As you suggest, the community aspect of these apps could truly be a game changer. What if people could interact with each other the same way you do in forums? The current apps we have don't allow for that kind of interaction. Instead, I end up feeling isolated, confined to a solitary interface without the ability to engage with others.

(CARMEN) Yeah, that's the essence of it. Capitalism operates by enclosing and privatising the commons. With the rise of techno-capitalism, this process has been accelerated. After all, the commons, the public sphere, and even data—a collectively generated resource—have all become commodities. There is no singularity; instead, there are just vast quantities of information and bodies, forming a collective network. However, this solidarity model is then enclosed and exploited, following the historical pattern of capitalism. It seizes upon the social bonds, fractures them, and causes profound trauma.

(MORGANE) How ironic that platforms such as Facebook, Reddit, and YouTube have, in a strange way, facilitated the resurgence of online gatherings and rituals, particularly among women. Historically, societal institutions like the Church often discouraged or suppressed such gatherings. They were dismissed as peculiar or mystical practices. However, now they have found a home on the internet. The irony lies in the fact that while these apps exist, you can nowadays only interact with an AI and not with other individuals to share your thoughts and experiences. We've been given the option to share experiences, but have to interact with an artificial being.

(CARMEN) We do need to revisit the tragedy of the commons, a concept that sits at the heart of capitalism. This idea suggests that when a resource is commonly available, someone will inevitably attempt to monopolise it, depriving others of access. This tragedy is evident in the realm of sociality, information, and data. In the 1990s, the internet held immense promise and excitement, with the potential to become a powerful platform for political engagement. However, during the Web 2.0 era, I vividly recall a conference where Jeff Bezos articulated the need to develop a business model centred around capturing attention as a means to generate profits through participation. This marked the moment when the tragedy of the commons unfolded: the moment someone took hold of the collective resource, thus severing the means for everyone to benefit from it. We need to move beyond data anxiety and see data as what it should be, namely, a publicly owned commodity.

(MORGANE) What would you imagine an ideal platform to look like, one that combines feminist principles and the commons?

(CARMEN) We have to collaborate with designers on this. I have my visions and ideas regarding the visual representation of this platform. Firstly, we would completely dismantle these wellness typology tropes that assume a 'perfect', 'seamless', glitch-free experience. Taking cues from the aestheticapproaches suggested by thinkers such as Legacy Russel, the intention, or rather assumption, would be that of the incalculable, the contingent. I'm not a designer myself, but I would love to discuss this in more detail with interface design thinkers to talk about how this intention could really come into play in a functional sense. There are definitely more 'choices', more options, perhaps a notification asking how many hours have you worked today? Different intentions or instrumentalisations of data. An alternative to pods of techno-capitalist 'salvation' where subjects are actually entirely isolated, alone. We must embrace our imagination and explore new aesthetics as we jump into this endeavour.

(MORGANE) Would such an app be decentralised? Would it be open-source? How would the community aspect take shape?

(CARMEN) I imagine it to resemble internet-based public housing in terms of appearance. It wouldn't necessarily have loads of visual appeal or 'sexy' aesthetics, but rather prioritise a functionality that promotes user engagement and provides accessible choices. Consider the architecture of public housing in Vienna as a reference point. It's like walking through the Karl Marx Hof in Vienna, and I envision a design interface that captures this. The challenge lies in determining its equivalent in the realm of digital design.

(MORGANE) Could such a platform be state-owned? A common market doesn't currently exist in the world. Therefore, why would we expect health apps, for instance, to adhere to such a planetary model? Does this mean the platform would be limited to a national scale, with separate state-owned entities in each country following their specific regulations? For instance, India might have different approaches to health systems than the United States.

(CARMEN) Maybe the platform could operate within an anarcho-syndicalist model, which was proposed by Elinor Ostrom and won the Nobel Peace Prize in Economic Science. Ostrom's model outlines an approach that manages property without a central authority. Essentially, it proposes the idea of scale, and mediation of scale via networks as the key to forming commons. So no, maybe it shouldn't be state-owned. But perhaps the data generated from the app could become a communally owned and

communally instrumentalised commodity on a smaller scale, and afterwards distributed and exchanged across a wider network.

(MORGANE) And given this complexity of creating a universal critical understanding of those apps, how does this conversation continue to progress and maintain criticality? Who is there to hold accountable for unsafe spaces, misleading pieces of information, and hyper-normative designs?

(CARMEN) My two cents: we need to keep emphasising that the issues at hand are structure, intention, plus how technology or design relates to these structural intentions. Of course, these technologies exist in a dialectical relationship with these structures, but I think we really need to collaborate with each other to imagine what new technologies and designs could look like; otherwise, we're stuck in the pitfall of having 'no alternative'. To quote Bernadette Krejs' recent PhD on housing, maybe we need to imagine FemTech otherwise, a re-imagining just like with housing: where it's not about removing the need for it, but instead centring ourselves on this otherwise. All the potential things that could be.

(MORGANE) Truly a thing to look forward to. Carmen, thank you so much for this conversation, and for being such a great collaborator and friend.

Acknowledge-ments

This project and its whole process would have never been possible without the infinite and unconditional support of Geert Lovink, Chloë Arkenbout and Laurence Scherz at the Institute of Network Cultures.

Thanks to Juli Frodermann, who accompanied me during an integral part of this project, giving me the space to be radical in both my ideas and my body. I know that loving me wasn't easy.

The list of individuals who helped me and inspired me is endless, but those who will read this text and who have been part of my life these past two years will easily recognise themselves. Thank you all.

Bibliography

Books

Amoore, Louise, and Volha Piotukh (eds.). *Algorithmic Life: Calculative Devices in the Age of Big Data*. London: Routledge, 2016.

Apprich, Clemens, Florian Cramer, Wendy Hui Kyong Chun, and Hito Steyerl. *Pattern Discrimination*. Minnesota: University of Minnesota Press, 2018.

Boyer, Anne. *The Undying: A Meditation on Modern Illness*. New York: MacMillan, 2019.

D'Ignazio, Catherine, and Lauren F. Klein. *Data Feminism*. Cambridge: MIT Press, 2023.

Enright, Lynn. *Vagina: A Re-Education*. Bloomsbury: Atlantic Books, 2021.

Fausz, Aaron, and W. Terry Howell. Healthcare Is Killing Us: *The Power of Disruptive Innovation to Create a System That Cares More and Costs Less*. Nashville: Skye Solutions, 2019.

Finn, Ed. *What Algorithms Want: Imagination in the Age of Computing*. Cambridge: MIT Press, 2018.

Gay, Roxanne. *Not That Bad, Dispatches from Rape Culture*. New York: Harper Collins, 2018.

Gray, Miranda. *The Optimized Woman*. London: John Hunt Publishing, 2009.

Greenfield, Ben. *Boundless: Upgrade Your Brain, Optimize Your Body & Defy Aging*. Cleveland: Victory Belt Publishing, 2020.

Haraway, Donna. *A Cyborg Manifesto*. London: The Socialist Review, 1985.

Hauskeller, Michael. *Mythologies of Transhumanism*. London: Palgrave Macmillan, 2016.

Hauskeller, Michael. *Sex and the Posthuman Condition*. London: Palgrave MacMillan, 2014.

Jackson, Gabrielle. Pain and Prejudice: *How the Medical System Ignores Women And What We Can Do About It*. Vancouver: Greystone Books, 2021.

Maté, Gabor, M.D. *Trauma, Illness, and Healing in a Toxic Culture*. London: EburyPublisher, 2022.

Preciado, Paul B. *Testo Junkie*. New York: Feminist Press, 2021.

Russell, Legacy. *Glitch Feminism*. London: Verso Books, 2020.

Sontag, Susan. *Illness as a Metaphor*. New York: Farrar Straus & Giroux, 1978.

Thornton, Cassie. *The Hologram*. Chicago: Pluto Press, 2020.

Tolentino, Jia. *Trick Mirror*. New York: Random House, 2019.

Ussher, Jane M. *Women and Madness, Myth and Experience*. London: Routledge Books, 2011.

Vitti, Alisa. WomanCode: *Perfect Your Cycle, Amplify Your Fertility, Supercharge Your Sex Drive, and Become a Power Source*. New York: Harper Collins, 2014.

Vries de, Glen, and Jeremy Blachman. *The Patient Equation: The Precision Medicine, Revolution in the Age of COVID-19 and Beyond*. New York: Wiley, 2020.

Wajcman, Judy. *Techno Feminism*. New York: Wiley, 1993.

Journal Articles and Theses

Ah-King, Malin, A.B. Barron, and M.E. Herberstein. "Genital Evolution: Why Are Females Still Understudied?" *PLOS Biology* 12, no. 5 (2011): 1001851. https://doi.org/10.1371/journal.pbio.1001851.

Ancker, Jessica S., Kristen M. Carpenter, Paul Greene, Randi Hoffman, Rita Kukafka, Laura A. V. Marlow, Holly G. Prigerson, and John M. Quillin. "Peer-to-Peer Communication, Cancer Prevention, and the Internet." *Journal of Health Communication* 14 Suppl 1, no. 0 1 (2009): 38–46. https://doi.org/10.1080/10810730902806760.

Baden-Fuller, Charles, and Stefan Haefliger. "Business Models and Technological Innovation." *Long Range Planning* 46 (2013): 419–26.

Beer, David. "Power Through the Algorithm? Participatory Web Cultures and the Technological Unconscious." *New Media & Society* 11 (September 7, 2009): 985–1002. https://doi.org/10.1177/1461444809336551.

Bleicken, Benjamin, Stefanie Hahner, Manfred Ventz, and Marcus Quinkler. "Delayed Diagnosis of Adrenal Insufficiency Is Common: A Cross-Sectional Study in 216 Patients." *The American Journal of the Medical Sciences* 339, no. 6 (June 2010): 525–31. https://doi.org/10.1097/MAJ.0b013e3181db6b7a.

Bresnahan, Mary Jiang, and Lisa Murray-Johnson. "The Healing Web." *Health Care for Women International* 23, no. 4 (June 1, 2002): 398–407. https://doi.org/10.1080/0739933029008964.

Catlaw, Thomas J., and Billie Sandberg. "The Quantified Self and the Evolution of Neoliberal Self-Government: An Exploratory Qualitative Study." *Administrative Theory & Praxis* 40, no. 1 (2018): 3-22.https://doi.org/10.1080/10841806.2017.1420743.

Chen, Zhiyi, Ziyao Wang, Meng Du, and Zhenyu Liu. "Artificial Intelligence in the Assessment of Female Reproductive Function Using Ultrasound: A Review." *Journal of Ultrasound in Medicine* 41, no. 6 (June 1, 2022): 1343–53. https://doi.org/10.1002/jum.15827.

Chrisler, Joan C., and Paula Caplan. "The Strange Case of Dr. Jekyll and Ms. Hyde: How PMS Became a Cultural Phenomenon and a Psychiatric Disorder." *Annual Review of Sex Research* 13 (2002): 274–306.

Corbin, Bethany. "Digital Micro-Aggressions and Discrimination: FemTech and the 'Othering' of Women." *Nova Law Review*, Vol. 44, 2020, 2020. https://ssrn.com/abstract=3630435.

DeCook, Julia. "A [White] Cyborg's Manifesto: The Overwhelmingly Western Ideology Driving Technofeminist Theory." *Media, Culture & Society* 43 (2020): 016344372095789. https://doi.org/10.1177/0163443720957891.

Eghaneyan, Brittany H., Katherine Sanchez, and Diane B. Mitschke. "Implementation of a Collaborative Care Model for the Treatment of Depression and Anxiety in a Community Health Center: Results from a Qualitative Case

Study." *Journal of Multidisciplinary Healthcare* 7 (2014): 503–13. https://doi.org/10.2147/JMDH.S69821.

Feng, Qizhang and Du, Mengnan and Zou, Na and Hu, Xia. "Fair Machine Learning in Healthcare: A Review." *ArXiv*, 2022. https://doi.org/10.48550/arxiv.2206.14397.

Figueroa, Caroline A., M.D., Tiffany Luo, MSW, Adrian Aguilera, PhD, and Courtney R Lyles, PhD. "The Need for Feminist Intersectionality in Digital Health." *The Lancet* Volume 3, Issue 8 (August 2021), https://www.thelancet.com/journals/landig/article/PIIS2589-7500(21)00118-7/fulltext.

Fumagalli, Andrea, Stefano Lucarelli, Elena Musolino, and Giulia Rocchi. "Digital Labour in the Platform Economy: The Case of Facebook." *Sustainability* 10, no. 6 (2018). https://doi.org/10.3390/su10061757.

Hendl, Tereza, and Bianca Jansky. "Tales of Self-Empowerment through Digital Health Technologies: A Closer Look at 'Femtech.'" *Review of Social Economy* 80, no. 1 (January 2, 2022): 29–57. https://doi.org/10.1080/00346764.2021.2018027.

Hoffman, Ginger A., and Jennifer L. Hansen. "Is Prozac a Feminist Drug?" *International Journal of Feminist Approaches to Bioethics* 4, no. 1 (2011): 89-120,. https://doi.org/10.2979/intjfemappbio.4.1.89.

Igoe, Katherine J. "Algorithmic Bias in Health Care Exacerbates Social Inequities — How To Prevent It." *Harvard School of Public Health* (blog), March 12, 2021. https://www.hsph.harvard.edu/ecpe/how-to-prevent-algorithmic-bias-in-health-care/.

Kapp, Marshall B. "Introduction: Law and Aging." *Journal of Law, Medicine and Ethics* 18, no. 3 (1990): 181–82.

Kim, Hun-Sung, Dai-Jin Kim, and Kun-Ho Yoon. "Medical Big Data Is Not Yet Available: Why We Need Realism Rather than Exaggeration." *Endocrinol Metab* (Seoul), 2019. https://doi.org/doi:10.3803/EnM.2019.34.4.349.

Kruse, Scott Clemens, Rishi Goswamy, Yesha Raval, and Sarah Marawi. "Challenges and Opportunities of Big Data in Health Care: A Systematic Review." *JMIR Medical Informatics* 4, no. 4 (2016).

Lekadir, Karim. "Artificial Intelligence in Healthcare. Applications, Risks, and Ethical and Societal Impacts." University of Barcelona Department of Mathematics and Computer Science, Artificial, Intelligence in Medicine Lab, Barcelona, Spain. May 2022. https://www.europarl.europa.eu/RegData/etudes/STUD/2022/729512/EPRS_STU(2022)729512_EN.pdf.

Leys, Colin. "Health, Health Care and Capitalism." *Socialist Register* 46 (2009): 1–28.

Loftus, Tyler, J. Patrick J. Tighe, Tezcan Ozrazgat-Baslanti, John P. Davis, Matthew M. Ruppert. "Ideal Algorithms in Healthcare: Explainable, Dynamic, Precise, Autonomous, Fair, and Reproducible." *PLOS Digital Health*, January 18, 2022. January 18, 2022.

Masri, Azza El. "Body Perfect in a Capitalist World: An Analysis of Consumer Culture and The Perfect Body Image." *Research Paper*, April 22, 2013.

McKee, Janet. "Holistic Health and the Critique of Western Medicine." *Social Science & Medicine* 26, no. 8 (January 1, 1988): 775–84, https://doi.org/10.1016/0277-9536(88)90171-2.

McKelvey, Fenwick, and Joshua Neves, eds. "Introduction: Optimization and Its Discontents." Review of Communication 21, no. 2 (2021): 95-112, https://doi.org/10.1080/15358593.2021.1936143.

National Institutes of Health. "Sex Hormone-Sensitive Gene Complex Linked to Premenstrual Mood." January 3, 2017. https://www.nih.gov/news-events/news-releases/sex-hormone-sensitive-gene-complex-linked-premenstrual-mood-disorder.

Newcastle University Press Office. "Fertility Apps with Millions of Users Collect and Share Excessive Data." May 4, 2021. https://www.ncl.ac.uk/press/articles/archive/2021/05/fertilityapps/.

Pilver, Corey, E. "Exposure to American Culture Is Associated with Premenstrual Dysphoric

Disorder among Ethnic Minority Women." *Journal of Affective Disorders* 130, 1-2 (2011): 334–41. https://doi.org/10.1016/j.jad.2010.10.013.

Roetman, Sara. "Self-Tracking 'Femtech': Commodifying & Disciplining the Fertile Female Body." *AoIR Selected Papers of Internet Research* 2020, no. 21 (October 5, 2020). https://doi.org/10.5210/spir.v2020i0.11320.

Siapka, Anastasia, and Elisabetta Biasin. 2021."“Bleeding Data: The Case of Fertility and Menstruation Tracking Apps." *Internet Policy Review* 10 (4). https://doi.org/10.14763/2021.4.1599.

Sik, Domonkos. "From Lay Depression Narratives to Secular Ritual Healing: An Online Ethnography of Mental Health Forums." *Culture, Medicine, and Psychiatry* 45, no. 4 (December 1, 2021): 751–74. https://doi.org/10.1007/s11013-020-09702-5.

Sysling, Fenneke. "Measurement, Self-Tracking and the History of Science: An Introduction." History of Science 58, no. 2 (July 1, 2020): 103–16. https://doi.

org/10.1177/0073275319865830.

Tran, Thi Ngoc Trang, Alexander Felfernig, Christoph Trattner, and Andreas Holzinger. "Recommender Systems in the Healthcare Domain: State-of-the-Art and Research Issues." Journal of Intelligent Information Systems 57, no. 1 (August 1, 2021): 171–201. https://doi.org/10.1007/s10844-020-00633-6.

Ussher, Jane M. "The Ongoing Silencing of Women in Families: An Analysis and Rethinking of Premenstrual Syndrome and Therapy." *Journal of Family Therapy* 25, no. 4 (2003): 388-405. Accessed June 10, 2023. https://doi.org/10.1111/1467-6427.00257.

Van Dijck, José. "Datafication, Dataism, and Dataveillance: Big Data Between Scientific Paradigm and Ideology." *Surveillance & Society* 12 (May 9, 2014): 197–208. https://doi.org/10.24908/ss.v12i2.4776.

Magazine and Online Articles

Cao, Patric. "Flo Health: Big Data in 'FemTech.'" *Harvard Edu* (blog), October 3, 2022. https://d3.harvard.edu/platform-digit/submission/flo-health-big-data-in-femtech/#:~:text=Flo%20Health%20is%20building%20and,sensitive%20personal%20reproductive%20health%20data/.

Downey-Mavromatis, Arminda. "No Ethical Vitamin Consumption Under Capitalism." *Columbia Spectator*, September 25, 2018. https://www.columbiaspectator.com/the-eye/2018/09/25/no-ethical-vitamin-consumption-under-capitalism/.

Elliott, Vittoria. "Fertility and Period Apps Can Be Weaponized in a Post-Roe World." *Wired*, June 7, 2022. https://www.wired.com/story/fertility-data-weaponized/.

Fair, Lesley. "Health App Broke Its Privacy Promises by Disclosing Intimate Details about Users." *Federal Trade Commission*, January 13, 2021. https://www.ftc.gov/business-guidance/blog/2021/01/health-app-broke-its-privacy-promises-disclosing-intimate-details-about-users.

Hull, Megan. "Premenstrual Dysphoric Disorder Statistics." In *The Recovery Village Blog*, 2023. https://www.therecoveryvillage.com/mental-health/pmdd/pmdd-statistics/.

Kraft, Oriana. "FemTech Startups Innovating Hormonal Health." *FemTechnology*, March 24, 2022. https://femtechnology.org/2022/03/24/femtech-startups-innovating-hormonal-health/.

Kung, Sidney. "Adapting Data Science for Non-Binary Inclusivity." *Towards Data Science*, 2020. https://towardsdatascience.com/adapting-data-science-for-non-binary-inclusivity-368f35a560e3.

Lacina, Anastasia. "Sexism Kills: Medical Misogyny and Ignorance of Female Bodies." *Fordham Political Review*, 2019. http://fordhampoliticalreview.org/sexism-kills-medical-misogyny-and-ignorance-of-female-bodies/.

Leisner, Amy, and Marissa Pomerance. "This Disorder Affects Millions Of Women, And No One Is Talking About It. Why?" *The Candidly*, 2021. https://www.thecandidly.com/2019/pmdd-affect-millions-of-women-so-why-arent-we-talking-about-it/.

Lucey, Kate. "PMDD Is the Condition That Means Your Period Can Make You Suicidal." *Metro*, 2019. https://metro.co.uk/2019/10/05/pmdd-condition-means-period-can-make-suicidal-10865751/.

Magistretti, Bérénice. "Flo Raises $5 Million for Its AI-Powered Period-Tracking App." *Venture Beat*, August 11, 2017. https://venturebeat.com/entrepreneur/flo-raises-5-million-for-its-ai-powered-femtech-app/.

Mayer, Beth Ann. "Complementary and Alternative Medicine Is Becoming Less 'Alternative' – Here's Why." *Healthline*, May 19, 2021. https://www.healthline.com/health/why-more-people-are-turning-to-complementary-and-alternative-medicine/.

Nadis, Steve. "The Downside of Machine Learning in Health Care." *News MIT*, February 1, 2022. https://news.mit.edu/2022/marzyeh-ghassemi-explores-downside-machine-learning-health-care-0201#:~:text=Even%20mechanical%20devices%20can%20contribute,for%20people%20with%20darker%20skin/.

Newcastle University. "Many Fertility Apps Not Exactly Fussy about Data Privacy, Study Shows." *Health Care In Europe*, July 5, 2021. https://healthcare-in-europe.com/en/news/many-fertility-apps-not-exactly-fussy-about-data-privacy-study-shows.html/.

News Desk. "Watch Now: Femtech Roundtable 2022 Can We Bridge the Gender Health Gap?" *FemTech World*, 2023. https://www.femtechworld.co.uk/special/watch-now-femtech-roundtable-2022-can-we-bridge-the-gender-health-gap/.

NIH. "NIH Inclusion Outreach Toolkit: How to Engage, Recruit, and Retain Women in Clinical Research." n.d. https://orwh.od.nih.gov/toolkit/recruitment/history/.

Renault, Marion. "No One Has to Get Their Period Anymore." *The Atlantic*, July 23, 2020. https://www.theatlantic.com/science/archive/2020/07/why-menstruate-if-you-dont-have/614350/.

Rigg, Kirsty. "How AI Can Empower Women's Health." *HT World*, August 31, 2022. https://www.htworld.co.uk/news/how-ai-can-empower-womens-health/.

"R/PMDD." Reddit Channel, n.d. https://www.reddit.com/r/PMDD/.

Saba, Vanessa. "The Human Experience Will Not Be Quantified." *New York Times*, 2020. https://www.nytimes.com/2020/11/07/opinion/sunday/data-science-limits.html/.

SciLifeLab. "Machine Learning Classifies Premenstrual Dysphoric Disorder in Terms of Grey Matter Structure." *SciLifeLab*, November 9, 2022. https://www.scilifelab.se/news/machine-learning-classifies-premenstrual-dysphoric-disorder-in-terms-of-grey-matter-structure/.

Scott, Jody. "Fake Periods, Side Effects, and Other Things You Need to Know about the Pill". *Vogue Australia*, 2018. https://www.vogue.com.au/beauty/wellbeing/fake-periods-side-effects-and-other-things-you-need-to-know-about-the-pill/news-story/006e70f2afb4fd78c4616bcd1417add2/.

Stewart, Conor. "Artificial Intelligence (AI) in Healthcare Market Size Worldwide from 2021 to 2030." *Statista*, September 28, 2022. https://www.statista.com/statistics/1334826/ai-in-health-care-market-size-worldwide/.

Wenner Moyer, Melinda. "Women Are Calling Out 'Medical Gaslighting'." *New York Times*, March 31, 2022. https://www.nytimes.com/2022/03/28/well/live/gaslighting-doctors-patients-health.html/.

Author biography

Morgane Billuart (1997) is a French writer and filmmaker. She completed her studies at the Gerrit Rietveld Academie in Amsterdam and also pursued education at the Cooper Union in New York. In an era dominated by digital culture, the enthusiasm for DIY internet philosophies, and the proliferation of self-help seminars, her distinctive approach seeks to shed light on the contemporary dynamics of faith and belief formation. Her work consistently grapples with these themes, intricately intertwined with her identity as a woman, prompting contemplation on the roles of bodies in reshaping the technocratic and digital landscapes that encompass us.

Colophon

Set Margins' #30

Cycles, The Sacred and The Doomed
Inquiries in Female Health Technologies
Morgane Billuart

First print January 2024
Second print January 2025

ISBN 978-90-833501-8-9

Editor:
Laurence Scherz
Chloë Arkenbout

Graphic design:
Winona Hudec

Text editor:
Laurence Scherz

Proofreader:
Laurence Scherz

Advisor:
Geert Lovink
Set Margins'

Fonts:
BB Baskervvol by
Typothèque Bye Bye Binary

PP Editorial New by
Pangram Pangram Foundry

Baskerville italic

Paper:
Munken Print Cream
15 100g (inside)
Munken Pure 200g (cover)

Printer:
Petro ofsetas

Made possible thanks to
the generous support of:
the Institute of Network Cultures

institute of
network cultures

and Stichting de Zaaier

STICHTING DE ZAAIER

Special thanks to friends, lovers,
relatives and Fiverr clients.

Set Margins'
www.setmargins.press